I0115383

CHOCOLATE AND THE NOBEL PRIZE

The Book of Brain Food

DR. CHONG CHEN

Brain & Life Publishing
London

ISBN 978-1-912533-01-5 Paperback

Brain & Life Publishing

27 Old Gloucester Street, London, U.K.

First Printing, 2018

For information about special needs for bulk purchases, sales promotions, and educational needs, please contact orders@brainandlife.net.

The Anchor of Our Purest Thoughts
Series

*1. Fitness Powered Brains: Optimize Your
Productivity, Leadership and Performance*

*2. Chocolate and the Nobel Prize: The Book of Brain
Food*

3. Cleverland: The Science of How Nature Nurtures

*4. The Tale of Two Minds: The Art and Science of
Decision-making in Everyday Life*

*5. Strategic Memory: The Natural History of Learning
and Forgetting*

To Arisa and my parents for their love and support

Yao Shi Tong Yuan [Medicine and food have the same roots].

—Ancient Chinese Saying

Let food be thy medicine.

—Hippocrates

Table of Contents

PART 1. FOOD FOR THOUGHT 1

Chapter 1. Introduction 2

Chapter 2. Chocolate, a Double-edged Sword 9

Chapter 3. Wine, or Grapes? 21

Chapter 4. The Benefit of 10 Cups of Green Tea 32

Chapter 5. Berry Everyday 39

Chapter 6. Olives, for Peace and (Cognitive) Power 45

Chapter 7. Nuts: Only Skin-deep? 51

Chapter 8. In Search of Coldwater, Fatty Fish 60

Chapter 9. The Healthy Way (1): From "5 A Day" to "10 A Day" 68

Chapter 10. The Healthy Way (2): The Mediterranean Diet .. 78

Chapter 11. The Unhealthy Way: 4 Driving Forces 86

Chapter 12. The Case for Dairy 94

Chapter 13. Spices, as Precious as Gold 100

PART 2. FOOD FOR FEELINGS AND SLEEP 105

Chapter 14. Mood-boosting Foods 106

Chapter 15. Foods That Help You Sleep 114

PART 3. CONCLUSION 121

Chapter 16. We Are What We Eat 122

REFERENCES.. 127

INDEX.. 197

ABOUT THE AUTHOR 203

PART 1. FOOD FOR THOUGHT

Chapter 1. Introduction

The beverage of the gods was Ambrosia; that of man is chocolate. Both increase the length of life in a prodigious manner.

— Louis Lewin, *Phantastica* (1924)

I do not like chocolate. More accurately, I hate chocolate. Years ago, I visited Los Angeles, where chocolate is exceptionally delicious and quite popular. So on the day of my return home, as a souvenir, I bought a lot of chocolate—a large container and a box of a famous brand—for my wife. She liked it very much. As chocolate contains many calories, we made a rule: one piece of chocolate a day. It took over two months for my wife to finish all the chocolate. During that period, we were very happy. She enjoyed the chocolate. I enjoyed her happiness.

Unfortunately, not long later, things changed. My wife noticed that her body weight had increased by three kilograms. *"Perhaps it was because of the chocolate,"* she thought. She started to complain about the chocolate, and me, who bought it for her. That's when I started to hate chocolate.

My story with chocolate didn't end there. Several months later, a report published in the *New England Journal of Medicine* came to my attention. Chocolate again, but this time, with positive outcomes.

Eat chocolate to win the Nobel Prize?

The report was authored by Dr. Franz H. Messerli, a physician working at St. Luke's–Roosevelt Hospital in New York. Dr. Messerli was a chocolate lover who claimed to eat chocolate every day. Extending his love for chocolate, Dr. Messerli looked at the yearly chocolate consumption per person in 23 countries all over the world. Then he did something extraordinary. He retrieved the number of the Nobel laureates in these countries until October 10, 2011 (the report was published in 2012) and checked if it related to chocolate consumption.

Surprisingly, Dr. Messerli found a statistically significant association. The more yearly chocolate consumption per person in one country, the higher the number of Nobel laureates per 10 million persons in that country. The correlational coefficient, a statistical marker measuring how good two variables change with each other, was as high as about 0.8. A correlational coefficient this big would make any scientist excited.

Switzerland had the highest yearly chocolate consumption (over 12 kg per person) and the number of Nobel laureates (about 33 per 10 million people), followed by the U.K., Norway, Denmark, and Austria. China scored the lowest in both (less than 1 kg per person, and 0 Nobel laureates), falling behind Japan, Portugal, Greece, and Brazil. The U.S. with the Netherlands, France, Finland and several other countries were in the middle. Dr. Messerli further estimated that the minimum yearly chocolate amount necessary for a Nobel Prize is about 2 kg per person and that increasing yearly chocolate consumption by 400 g per person in a certain country could increase its number of Nobel laureates by one.

Chocolate for the Nobel Prize, seriously? This report has been controversial since its day of publication, as it is correlational and does not indicate causality. Some scientists even take it as a joke, since chocolate and Nobel Prizes seem far away from each other, and the correlation between them may come from a third, hidden factor. In line with this, a later report confirmed that the gross domestic product is a driver for both chocolate consumption and the number of Nobel laureates. The richer a country, the more likely its people are to eat chocolate. On the same note, the wealthier countries invest more in education and scientific research. And investment in education and scientific research is the main driver for the number of Nobel laureates.

Nevertheless, there does exist the possibility that eating chocolate may somehow increase people's chance of winning the Nobel Prize. Chocolate is made from cacao beans, which are rich in the chemical compounds flavanols. Flavanols are polyphenols, which enhance cognitive abilities (see Chapter 2). Therefore, the habit of eating chocolate may have helped the laureates lay the foundation of their award-winning work. Polyphenols also promote health and reduce the risk of chronic diseases, such as cardiovascular disease, diabetes, and cancer (see Chapter 2). Eating chocolate may have prolonged people's longevity and helped the Nobel laureates to get their prizes.

These two explanations assume that Nobel laureates actually do eat chocolate and more so than the average person. But do they? Being residents in a country where people tend to eat more chocolate does not guarantee the

Nobel laureates themselves eat more chocolate. If they never eat chocolate, then the story changes dramatically.

Are Nobel laureates more likely to eat chocolate?

A year after Dr. Messerli's research, another short report answering this question came out in the journal *Nature*. A team led by Dr. Beatrice A. Golomb at the University of California, San Diego actually surveyed 23 male winners of the Nobel Prize in physics, chemistry, physiology or medicine, and economics, and asked them how often they ate chocolate. The team then compared those results to another survey of 237 well-educated and age-matched male control subjects. It turned out that 10 of the Nobel laureates, or 43%, ate chocolate more than twice a week, while merely 25% of the control subjects did so. By statistical inference, this result indicates that the Nobel laureates are more likely than the average person to eat chocolate.

Here another question comes up. When did these Nobel laureates develop the habit of eating chocolate? If they developed it long before receiving their prize, chocolate might have contributed; but if they developed it after receiving the prize, this suggests that people with superior cognitive abilities are more likely to realize the benefit of chocolate and eat it more often. Unfortunately, the above study did not answer this question.

Anyway, being unable to answer this question did not bother my wife. She started to claim that, as she had eaten so much chocolate, all she had to do was to wait for the phone call from the Nobel Committee in Stockholm. To this day, the call has not come.

Chocolate for the Nobel Prize, seriously?

Eating chocolate promotes health and cognitive functions. People with better health and cognitive functions have a higher chance of winning the Nobel Prize. The logic behind the link is reasonable, although we do not know exactly how significant chocolate is for the Nobel Prize, especially in the face of many other, arguably more important, factors.

The Nobel Prize is a symbol of outstanding contribution to human society. It is embedded in our nature to seek excellence. We want to be higher, stronger, and faster, not only physically but also mentally. The attempt to link chocolate to the Nobel Prize reflects this ultimate pursuit of excellence. It is an exploration of the diet approach.

To date, thousands of studies have been conducted to investigate the effect of various foods on the mind. The results have been fruitful. The diet approach towards enhancing human performance has been one of the major approaches, besides physical exercise (see my book *Fitness Powered Brains*) and natural environment (see my book *CleverLand: How Nature Nurtures*).

Thus, this book is not about how to win the Nobel Prize but about which foods benefit the brain and how they help us think more effectively, feel more positively, and sleep more soundly. This book is a collection of brain foods identified by the scientific community. It is a synthesis of over 400 scientific reports published before December 2017.

So if you are reading this book because you want to win the Nobel Prize, sorry. But by consuming more brain foods and consuming them right, I am sure your chance of winning the Nobel Prize—any prize—will increase. Enjoy.

Chapter 2. Chocolate, a Double-edged Sword

Oh, comfortable cocoa!

— Dodie Smith,
I Capture the Castle (1949)

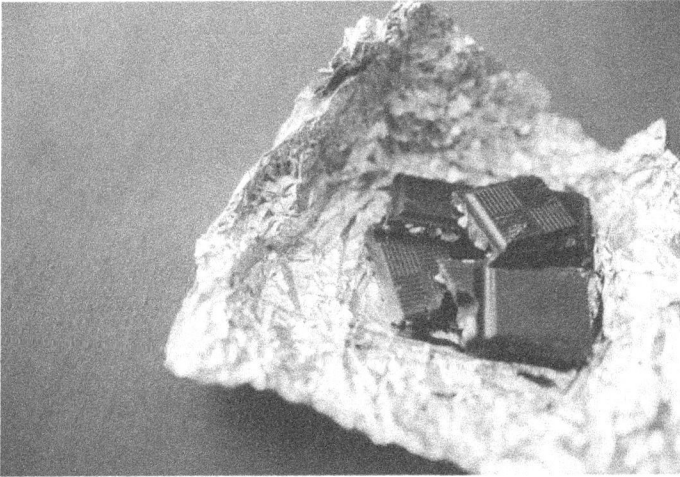

The health benefits of 2–3 servings of chocolate per week

Recently, two independent meta-analyses were published by Chinese researchers, reaching the same conclusion that chocolate, when consumed moderately, reduces the risk of chronic diseases. Scientists use meta-analysis to combine data from a large number of studies and identify a common effect. These two meta-analyses together included 19 surveys of over 600,000 subjects about their chocolate consumption and followed their health conditions until up to 16 years later.

The first meta-analysis estimated that the peak protective effect of chocolate consumption on chronic diseases occurred at two servings per week. One serving is typically defined as 30 g. Weekly two servings of chocolate reduced the risk of future diabetes by 25% and the risk of coronary heart disease and stroke by 10–16%. Consuming more chocolate conferred little additional benefit. In the second meta-analysis, one serving of chocolate per week reduced the risk of heart failure by 8%, three servings by 14%, while 7 and 10 servings had no benefit. These two meta-analyses suggest that eating a moderate amount of chocolate, namely about 2–3 servings per week, reduces the risk of chronic diseases.

Meanwhile, population-based surveys have also indicated the cognitive-enhancing effect of eating a moderate amount of chocolate. In a study of over 2,000 elderly people conducted by A. David Smith at the University of Oxford, U.K., those on average eating 2–3 servings of chocolate per week showed the highest performance in a battery of cognitive tests. The assumption that eating a moderate amount of chocolate may have assisted the previous Nobel laureates in getting their prizes is backed up by research.

Chocolate is made from cacao beans, which are rich in flavanols, such as epicatechin and catechin. Flavanols are polyphenols, a family of organic chemicals characterized by multiple phenol structural units. They naturally exist in plants and are produced by plants as defense mechanisms against environmental challenges, including ultraviolet radiation and pathogen attacks.

Excitingly, consuming foods rich in polyphenols also helps humans defend against environmental challenges. Over two decades of research suggest that polyphenols possess powerful, favorable effects on health. As diet affects the health of the body and brain through common biological pathways, both will be mentioned. The primary focus of this book, however, is on the brain.

The SOWING model of the brain

To conclude whether or not certain foods benefit the brain, we must use informative markers, be they behavioral or biological. Behavioral markers are more visible to the naked eye and measured by behavioral tasks such as an IQ or memory test. In contrast, biological markers are typically measured by laboratory assays such as a blood test. These informative markers are helpful in determining which foods are brain food and which are junk food, and what nutrients are to be praised or avoided.

For this purpose, I developed a simplified model of the brain, the "SOWING" model. SOWING are the initials of six informative markers:

- Stress hormones

- Oxidative stress

- Work performance

- Inflammation

- Neurons

- Growth factors

The six informative markers of SOWING represent six dimensions of the behavioral and biological aspects of our brain. As shown in the figure below, work performance is the behavioral output of the brain and the collective effect of the other five biological dimensions. Work performance reflects the efficiency and effectiveness of neurons and the neuronal network. Neurons and the neuronal network, in turn, are affected by stress hormones, oxidative stress, inflammation, and growth factors.

The SOWING model of the brain

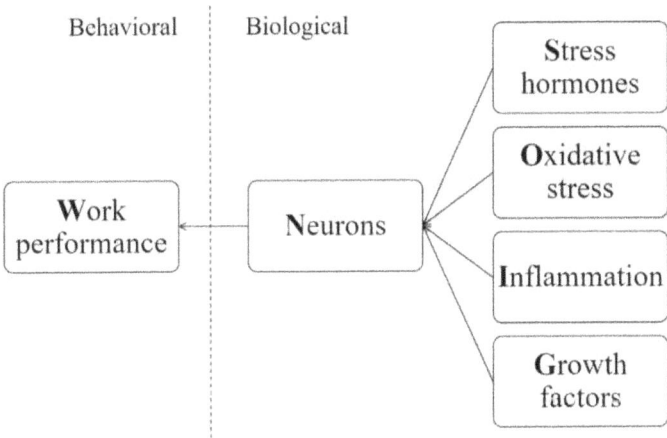

This model is based on my previous book, *The Seed of Intelligence: Boost Your Baby's Developing Brain through Optimal Nutrition and Healthy Lifestyle*, written for pregnant mothers, and originates from the analogy of sowing seeds to "grow" a more powerful brain—by improving our diet, for instance. For a brief introduction to these six dimensions, see the table below.

Table. The SOWING model of the brain

Sowing	Introduction
Stress hormones	Stress hormones are the products of the stress system or, more specifically, the hypothalamic-pituitary-adrenal axis. The final product and most well-known stress hormone is cortisol. Stress hormones are released to mobilize the body to deal with environmental challenges, such as physical injury and psychological stressors.
Oxidative stress	Oxidative stress arises when the production of free radicals—or reactive oxygen species (ROS)—exceeds the ability of the body to eliminate or neutralize them. ROS is the common outcome of normal cellular metabolism.
Work performance	Work performance here refers to primarily cognitive abilities, including the ability to memorize information (termed memory) and the ability to process information (executive function or working memory).
Inflammation	Inflammation is the immune system's response to harmful stimuli such as pathogens, in order to eradicate the harmful stimuli and protect the body. Upon activation of the immune system, pro-inflammatory cytokines are excreted from immune-related cells to promote inflammation and mediate the innate immune response.
Neurons	Neurons refer to the neuronal network and are the neurobiological basis of work performance (and all our mental experiences).
Growth factors	Growth factors are proteins synthesized in the body to promote the growth of cells including neurons.

Stress hormones, oxidative stress, and inflammation are normal reactions of the body to cope with environmental challenges, including physical injuries, infections, and psychological stressors, and to improve the chance of survival. However, too much of them are harmful to neurons, partly by reducing the level of growth factors. This can cause severe illness. High levels of stress hormones, oxidative stress, and inflammation indicate that the external environment is risky and/or the internal body status is unhealthy.

These six dimensions (stress hormones, oxidative stress, work performance, inflammation, neurons, and growth factors) are at the central stage of modern neuroscience; any other factor that affects the mind has its effect via one or several of these dimensions. We use these six dimensions together because they provide more information than each one separately, as neuroscientists in different fields tend to focus on different dimensions. For the purpose of reading this book, it is helpful to remember that SOWING is six informative markers used to differentiate brain food from junk food.

The "sowing" power of polyphenols

Research shows that polyphenols benefit the brain through all of the six dimensions of SOWING. Several weeks to months of treatment with polyphenols or food rich in polyphenols can:

- Reduce the release of **stress hormones** in response to environmental challenges (this relaxes us);

- Reduce **oxidative stress** by inhibiting and scavenging ROS and inhibiting pro-oxidant enzymes;

- Enhance **work performance**, including the ability to memorize information (e.g., word lists) and do logical reasoning, and prevent cognitive decline that typically occurs with aging;

- Reduce **inflammation** by blocking the synthesis of pro-inflammatory cytokines;

- Increase the production of **neurons** in the dentate gyrus of the hippocampus, a brain area responsible for encoding episodic memory (memory of elements and facts that comprise events), spatial navigation and emotion regulation;

- Increase the levels of **growth factors** such as brain-derived neurotrophic factor (BDNF), which supports the production, growth, differentiation, and survival of neurons.

In other words, polyphenols sow the seeds for our brain. Now we can see why chocolate is good for our brain and enhances cognitive functions.

Dark chocolate is better than white

Flavanols are the main form of polyphenols contained in chocolate and responsible for its benefits on the brain. Unfortunately, flavanols also give chocolate its bitter taste. As a result, chocolate makers often reduce the amount of flavanols. Worse, there is generally no information regarding the amount of flavanols on the labels of chocolate, making it hard to know how beneficial a particular piece of chocolate is (or is not).

However, one way to choose chocolate is by looking at its color. The darker the chocolate, the greater the proportion of cocoa solids (which contain flavanols), which increases the likelihood of a higher amount of flavanols.

A typical bar of dark chocolate contains about four times more flavanols than a milk chocolate bar, while white chocolate hardly has any. Meanwhile, it has been reported that milk proteins may bind to flavanols and interfere with the absorption of flavanols from dark chocolate. Consequently, choose dark chocolate over milk or white, and eat it without drinking milk or consuming another dairy.

The problem with chocolate

Chocolate is frequently categorized as a sweet. It contains much cocoa butter, a source of saturated fat, and often added sugar. Overeating chocolate causes excessive caloric intake and increases your chance of weight gain and obesity. Remember, this is what my wife had been complaining of and why I started to hate chocolate.

Worse, high consumption of saturated fat and obesity are harmful to the brain in all of the six dimensions of SOWING: they increase the level of stress hormones and oxidative stress, reduce work performance, increase inflammation, are toxic to neurons, and reduce growth factors. High levels of added sugar also increases oxidative stress and inflammation while impairing work performance.

Actually, chocolate, particularly milk chocolate, and other sweets are considered "comfort foods." High consumption of them characterizes a typical unhealthy diet. We will touch upon this topic in Chapter 11.

This major problem with chocolate explains why its peak benefit occurs with moderate consumption, namely around 2–3 servings per week.

Light brown natural cocoa can be consumed daily

Compared to chocolate, cocoa powder or cocoa contains less saturated fat as cocoa butter has been removed while retaining cocoa solids that contain flavanols. This allows cocoa to be consumed more frequently than chocolate, if it is sugar-free. Several well-conducted experiments have indicated the benefit of daily consumption of flavanol-rich cocoa drinks (e.g., 250 ml) on cognitive functions in young, middle-aged, and elderly adults.

Among commercially available cocoa powders, the preferred choice is natural cocoa powders, which contain more flavanols and typically are light brown in color. Flavanols taste bitter. The Dutching processing of cocoa power reduces this bitterness by alkalizing, which destroys flavanols, darkens the cocoa ingredient and increases the dispersibility for various beverages. The more heavily alkalized, the more decrease in flavanols. Therefore, natural cocoa powders are preferred to Dutched ones. But if natural cocoa powders are too bitter for you, opt for lightly Dutched cocoa powders, where roughly 40% of the natural level of flavanols is retained.

Chapter 3. Wine, or Grapes?

I went to an all-night get together

And everyone I knew was there.

Had the love that would last forever.

Everywhere I looked, I saw you standing there.

Get up; get your man a bottle of red wine.

— Eric Clapton, *Bottle of Red Wine* (1970)

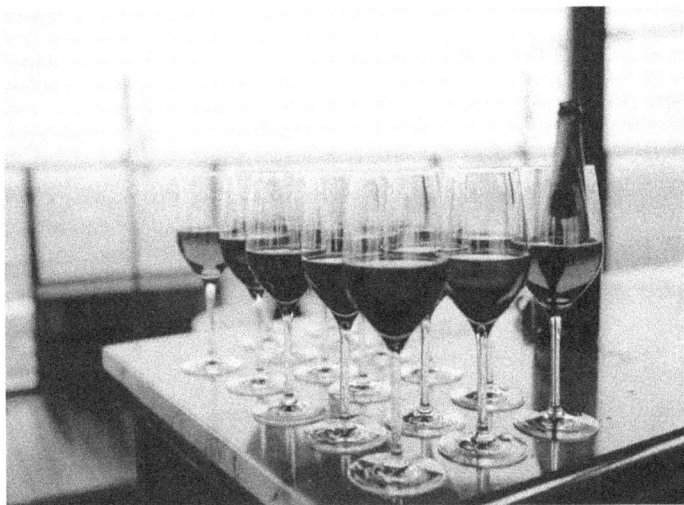

Professor Akito Kawaguchi (A.K.) was my first mentor in graduate school. He was tall, thin, walked fast, and had a bright and contagious personality. When A.K. visited Peking University Health Science Center, I went with him. It was during a cold winter. To my surprise, after getting to the hotel in the evening of the first day, he asked me to take him to the nearest supermarket. I thought he wanted some Chinese souvenirs and fortunately, there was one within a five minutes' walk. So we walked there, and A.K. bought a bottle of French red wine. It turned out that A.K. had the habit of drinking 1–2 glasses of red wine every day.

It was since then that I wondered about the effect of wine and other alcohols on health. A.K. is an expert in food and nutrition. He is a physician and health scientist specialized in lifestyle and chronic diseases. He led the *Sapporo Lifestyle Study* and was responsible for the annual health check of Kimobetsu Town residents for years. Both Sapporo and Kimobetsu Town are in Hokkaido, a northern island of Japan and where I received my Ph.D. in Medicine.

Indeed, the health benefit of wine first caught the eyes of scientists in the field of chronic diseases, specifically coronary heart disease (CHD). CHD, a cardiovascular disease, involves the narrowing of the coronary arteries that supply oxygen-rich blood to the heart. It is caused by the buildup of cholesterol and other waxy substances called plaque on the inner walls of the coronary arteries. Due to the reduced blood supply, the heart cannot get the blood or oxygen it needs. This often leads to chest pain, heart attacks, permanent heart damage, and ultimately death. Interestingly, those who drink a moderate amount of wine seem to have a lower risk of CHD.

"The French Paradox"

In 1992, Dr. Serge Renaud, a French scientist from Bordeaux, the world's major wine capital, published a report in the journal *Lancet*. This report was based on data from a worldwide disease monitoring project, *the Monitoring of Trends and Determinants on Cardiovascular Disease* (MONICA) organized by the World Health Organization.

Dr. Renaud found that the French, despite consuming a diet high in saturated fat, had a relatively low mortality rate of CHD compared to other countries. Saturated fat such as that in butter, cheese, fatty beef, lamb, and pork is a well-known risk factor for cardiovascular diseases. Nevertheless, the French presented about only one-third of the mortality compared to people in several other countries that consumed the same level of saturated fat, such as the

U.K., Denmark, Sweden, and Australia. This phenomenon has since been known as "The French Paradox."

In the same paper, a possible explanation of the paradox was attributed to the moderate daily consumption of red wine during French meals. It is estimated that the French on average drink 1–2 glasses of wine daily. Thus, Dr. Renaud argued that red wine is good for the heart. This theory soon became popular worldwide, and Dr. Renaud became a French hero.

Research done during the following two decades has supported this theory. Several large-scale prospective surveys estimated that moderate consumption of wine, namely 1–2 drinks a day, reduces the risk of mortality from all causes by 20–30%, cardiovascular disease by 10–30%, stroke by 30–40%, and the risk of cancer by 20%. One standard drink of wine is usually defined as 5 oz or 150 ml.

Low to moderate consumption of wine benefits cognitive ability

The benefit of wine applies to cognitive dimensions, too. One study followed almost 3,800 elderly people in the southwest part of France for three years. In these people, wine was the main alcoholic drink. It was found those with 1–2 drinks per day had 45% reduced risk of developing Alzheimer's disease, while those with 3–4 drinks per day had 72% reduced risk. Another Dutch study followed almost 8,000 people aged 55 years and above for six years and found that 1–3 drinks per day reduced the risk of developing dementia by 42%.

We know wine is more likely to be served at high-class restaurants. Doctors, lawyers, executives, and people with high socioeconomic status are more likely to drink a moderate amount of wine regularly. Meanwhile, surveys show that these moderate wine drinkers are more likely to be health conscious, to eat more fruits and vegetables, and to exercise more. So is the above observation a result of these confounding factors?

Surely not. Wine is an alcoholic beverage made from grapes, which contain rich polyphenols. Polyphenols, as we have seen, promote brain health through all of the six dimensions of SOWING. In the case of cognitive aging, the aggregation of amyloid beta-protein in the brain is believed to be a major driver for the cognitive decline including the development of dementia. Amyloid beta-protein aggregates in the extracellular areas of the brain and disrupts the membranes of neurons, leading to cognitive decline. Wine, through its rich polyphenols, can prevent the generation of amyloid beta-protein and attenuate, even reverse, the deterioration of cognitive functions. With CHD, polyphenols inhibit the oxidation of low-density lipoprotein, an important carrier of cholesterol. Consequently, polyphenol-rich wine can reduce the risk of CHD, which excellently explains the French Paradox.

Wine, rather than beer and spirits, is good

Although there have been sporadic reports that moderate amounts of alcohol promote health, prospective epidemiological studies overall support the benefit of moderate consumption of wine, but not beer or spirits. For instance, as shown by the *Canadian Study of Health and Aging* which followed up over 4,000 subjects, moderate consumption of wine reduced the risk of developing dementia in the 5-year follow-up period by 31%. In contrast, consumption of beer or spirits had no such benefit. This is in line with the fact that wine, but not beer or spirits, contains polyphenols.

Heavy drinking, irrespective of what one drinks, is bad

Nevertheless, research shows that alcohol (ethanol), especially when consumed in large amounts, such as heaving drinking or more than 3–4 drinks a day, is harmful to the brain.

- First, alcohol stimulates the secretion of **stress hormone** cortisol;

- Second, alcohol increases **oxidative stress** by decreasing antioxidant activity and increasing ROS production (because of alcohol metabolism in the liver);

- Third, alcohol impairs **work performance**. Alcohol reduces the ability of working memory to inhibit impulsive behavior. Heavy drinking also causes severe cognitive deficits and increases the risk of dementia;

- Fourth, alcohol increases pro-inflammatory cytokines and increases **inflammation** in the body;

- Fifth, alcohol induces abnormalities in glial cells; the latter provide nutrients to **neurons**. Alcohol also reduces the absorption of many nutrients especially vitamins like folate, thiamine, and B6, which are essential for the normal functioning of cells, including neurons. Thus, alcohol reduces neuronal survival and causes severe damage to the brain;

- Sixth, alcohol reduces the level of BDNF and inhibits the activity of insulin-like growth factor 1 (IGF-1). IGF-1 is another **growth factor** that promotes the growth of almost every cell in the body.

Thus, heavy drinking, irrespective of what alcoholic beverages one consumes, has toxic consequences in all of the six dimensions of SOWING.

Women are more susceptible to the harmful effects of alcohol

Compared to men, women on average have lower levels of the enzyme alcohol dehydrogenase, which metabolizes or breaks down alcohol. Women are more susceptible to the harmful effects of alcohol. Whereas two drinks per day is generally considered moderate in men, one is moderate in women. For your information, one standard drink is usually defined as 1.2 oz or 35 ml of spirits (such as gin, rum, tequila, vodka, and whiskey),

5 oz or 150 ml of wine, or 12 oz or 350 ml of beer (see figure below).

A standard drink

1.2 oz spirits	5 oz wine	12 oz beer

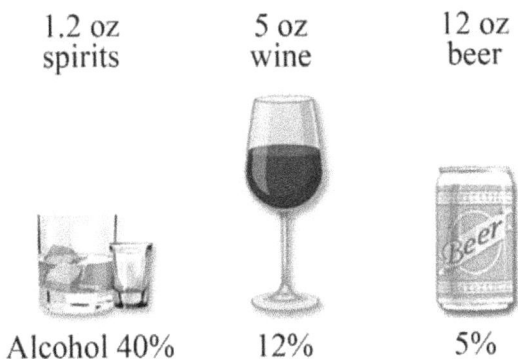

Alcohol 40%	12%	5%

Red wines are better than white ones

With moderate consumption of wine, the protective effect of polyphenols surpasses the detrimental effect of alcohol. That is why moderate consumption of wine benefits the brain. The balance between alcohol and polyphenols turns out to be critical.

Interestingly, it is estimated that red wines contain about 10-fold more polyphenols than their white counterparts. It is because red wines are fermented in the presence of seeds and skins while white is exclusively fermented by the grape juice only.

Polyphenols are richer in grape skins and seeds than in juice.

Red wine versus grapes, which to choose?

If the polyphenol component of red wine is good while the alcohol component is bad, then grapes, from which red wines are made, understandably, should be preferred. Meanwhile, grapes, grape juices, and dried grapes or raisins, contain many micronutrients such as vitamins and minerals, which are essential for the body and brain (see Chapter 9). For instance, research suggests that grape juices have a similar level of antioxidant potential and possess a superior inhibiting effect on the buildup of cholesterol compared to wines.

But we drink red wines not only because of their health benefits, but also because of their social and cultural meaning. Wines create romantic and festive atmospheres. Wines and other alcohols are typically indispensable at parties and in the celebration of important events. This social and cultural significance is unmatched by grapes, grape juices, or raisins. The same is true for chocolate, a symbol of love and romance. So what we can do is make the right choice at the right time to generate the optimal outcomes, both personal and social.

Finally, due to severe harmful effects, infants, toddlers, children, adolescents, and pregnant women should not drink any alcohol, while women and men trying to conceive should also restrain from alcohol (see my book *Before You Get Pregnant*).

Chapter 4. The Benefit of 10 Cups
of Green Tea

There are few hours in life more agreeable
than the hour dedicated to the ceremony
known as afternoon tea.

— Henry James, *The Portrait of a Lady* (1881)

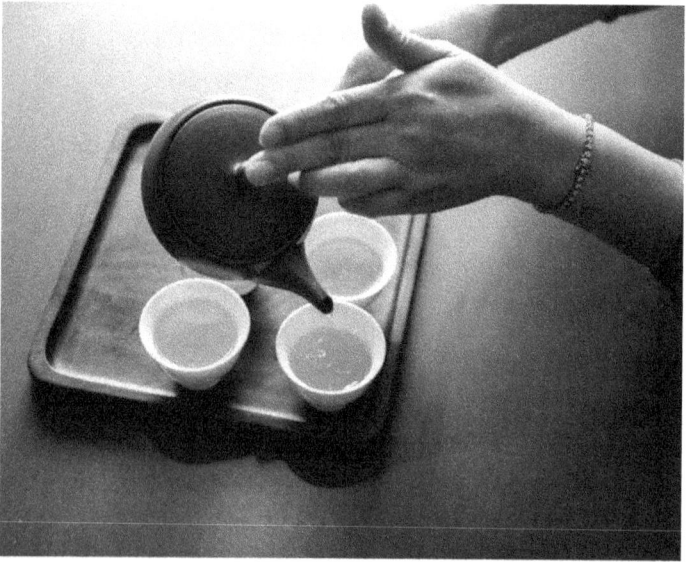

Green tea for cancer

Years ago, Keiko's husband John was diagnosed with colon cancer. He was told to have a survival chance of only 50%. Keiko didn't understand what exactly that figure meant, but she decided to do something to save her husband's life. Green tea came to her mind. Tea has been used in traditional Chinese medicine for over 4,000 years, and Keiko was born and raised in Japan, where traditional Chinese medicine is widely used and people believe in the health benefits of drinking tea. Several years earlier, a group of Japanese scientists had just reported that daily consumption of 10 cups of green tea reduces the risk and delays the onset of cancer.

Keiko told John (an American) to drink 10 cups of freshly brewed green tea every day. After some research, she chose sencha, a type of green tea that contains more polyphenols but less caffeine compared to other types of green tea such as matcha. John and his oncologist (who didn't know the benefit of green tea yet) didn't expect much from drinking this green tea. But John kept on drinking sencha. As time passed, John's cancer eventually showed improvement. Five years later, his oncologist told him that he had recovered from cancer and what he had to do from then on was to keep on drinking his green tea. The oncologist finally noticed the increasing scientific reports on the benefit of green tea on cancer. The antioxidant and anti-inflammatory effects of polyphenols are the main mechanism of cure.

Keiko and John's personal experience dramatically increased their passion towards green tea. After that, they created a company to provide green tea and share their story with the American public.

Tea benefits cognitive functions

A typical cup of brewed green tea is made with 2 g tea leaves immersed in 200 ml hot water. It contains about 500–700 mg of water-extractable materials, of which 30–40% (by dry weight) are catechin polyphenols such as epigallocatechin gallate. As we have explained the protective effects of polyphenols on the six dimensions of SOWING, here we introduce the benefit of green tea in regards to work performance.

The first epidemiological report of the neuroprotective effect of tea came from a 2002 study of 210 patients with Parkinson's disease and 347 healthy subjects living in Washington State, USA. It was estimated that daily consumption of two or more cups of tea reduced the risk of developing Parkinson's disease by 60%.

In another 2009 report from the *Hordaland Health Study* in Norway involving over 2,000 elderly people, the association between the consumption of tea (with black tea being the most common) and the performance on a battery of cognitive tests was linear. The more cups of tea drank every day, the better the cognitive performance. Notably, the greatest tea consumption among this population was five cups a day.

Regarding the type, any tea, be it green, black, or oolong, is beneficial. Nevertheless, the neuroprotective effect of green tea is the biggest.

Why green tea is better than black and oolong tea

Black and oolong tea is produced via fermentation, in which tea leaves are crushed to promote enzymatic oxidation and subsequent condensation of catechins polyphenols. The amount of polyphenols is lower in black and oolong (3–10% of the water-extractable material) compared to green tea (30–40%), while the amount of caffeine in them is similar (2–5% of the water-extractable material). This explains the superior health-promoting effect of green tea.

The caffeine concern of green tea

Tea contains caffeine, as does coffee, energy drinks, some soft drinks (such as colas), cocoa, and chocolate. At moderate doses, caffeine exerts stimulatory effects by blocking adenosine receptors in the brain in particular the cerebral cortex, hippocampus, and cerebellum. However, over-stimulation of neurons is toxic and may cause neuronal death.

According to *The 2015–2020 Dietary Guidelines for Americans* created by the U.S. Department of Health and Human Services, the daily allowance of the consumption of caffeine is 400 mg. This amount is typically contained in about 2–3 12-oz (350 ml) cups of drip/brewed or instant coffee, 10 cups of black tea, or 12–30 cups of green tea. Caffeine seems not a serious concern for drinking traditionally brewed green tea if you don't consume much coffee and other caffeine-rich drinks in general.

In addition, although chocolate and cocoa contain caffeine, the amount is about 4–7 times less than that in green tea, so there is little worry of overconsumption of caffeine if you consume both.

Coffee is better restricted

Coffee is a frequently consumed stimulant drink and an indispensable part of modern culture. Although there have been reports indicating that moderate consumption of coffee (2–3 cups a day) may reduce mortality and prevent cognitive decline, overall the evidence is limited and mixed. *The 2015–2020 Dietary Guidelines for Americans* concludes that moderate consumption of coffee is not associated with increased risk of chronic diseases, yet, individuals who do not drink coffee or other caffeinated beverages are not encouraged to acquire the habit.

Meanwhile, research indicates that high consumption of coffee is consistently harmful to health. Drinking five 8-oz (about 250 ml) cups of coffee containing approximately 500 mg of caffeine in total at one sitting produces a typical episode of stress response. In the *Italian Longitudinal Study on Aging*, elderly adults who increased their coffee drinking—even by merely one cup per day—during the 3.5-year study period had a higher risk of mild cognitive impairment.

Thus, if you do not drink coffee frequently, keep that habit. If you drink coffee every day, drink it moderately, no more than 2–3 cups.

Why green tea is so special

Green tea is special because its benefit is linear. The more we drink, the greater benefit we get. Whereas red wine and dark chocolate should be consumed only moderately, green tea can be safely consumed in large amounts between meals by most people (allergy is rare). Furthermore, the concentration of polyphenols in green tea is higher than that in red wine, dark chocolate, and cocoa drinks. In my own case, I usually drink 2–3 cups of green tea in the morning, 3–4 in the afternoon, and 2–3 cups in the evening.

Chapter 5. Berry Everyday

Strawberry Fields is anywhere you want to go.

— John Lennon

If you keep my secret, this strawberry is yours.

— Tsugumi Ohba

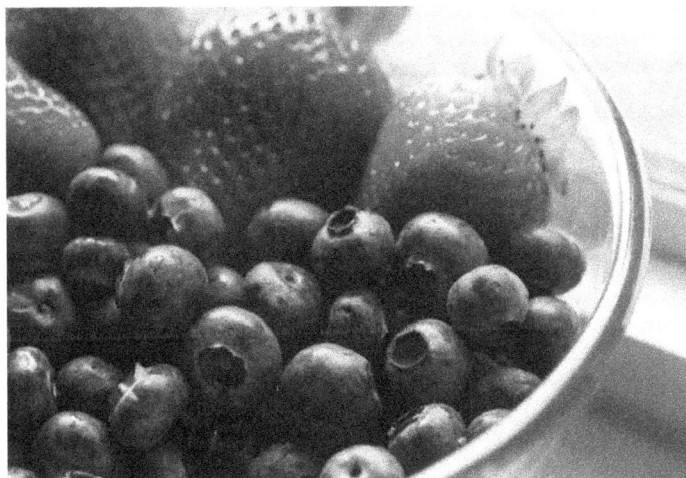

Berries enhance cognitive functions

Starting in 1980, over 120,000 nurses aged 30–55 years participated in the *Nurses' Health Study* conducted by researchers at Harvard Medical School. Every four years they were asked their diet habits in details, for instance, how often they ate each food. Between 1995 and 2001, more than 16,000 of them received cognitive tests and were followed up twice at two-year intervals after that. Statistical analysis indicated that after adjusting potential confounding factors such as age and educational background, greater consumption of blueberries and strawberries across the study period was associated with slower rates of cognitive decline. Specifically, it was estimated that the effect size of weekly two or more servings of strawberries (one serving is about 8 large strawberries) was equivalent to the delaying of about 1.5 years of cognitive aging. The effect size of weekly one or more servings of blueberries (one serving is about 75 g or 2.6 oz) was equivalent to the delaying of about 2 years of cognitive aging.

Berry is another brain food. Eating berries or drinking berry juice for merely several weeks has been found to improve cognitive functions. In one experiment conducted by researchers at the University of Cincinnati, elderly people with mild cognitive impairment showed marked improvement in cognitive functions after drinking blueberry juice every day for 12 weeks. They became better at remembering word lists and associative learning. Associative learning is essential for forming episodic memory, namely linking elements and facts that comprise events together. After drinking blueberry juice for 12 weeks, these elderly individuals also showed reduced depressive symptoms and lower blood glucose. In this study, the amount of daily juice was about 6–9 ml per kg body weight, which equals to 360–540 ml (12–18 oz) per day for an average person with a body weight of 60 kg or 132 pounds.

In another experiment conducted by researchers at Lund University, Sweden, drinking a 450 g mixed berry beverage every day for 5 weeks improved verbal working memory in healthy adults aged 50–70 years. Verbal working memory is the ability to process verbal information (e.g., identify nouns) while holding sentences in mind. It is a critical component of fluid intelligence, or the ability to make inferences and solve problems.

Berries are among the highest-ranked antioxidants

Berries, including strawberries, blueberries, blackberries, blackcurrant, cranberries, elderberry, lingonberries, chokeberries, and raspberries, are among the highest-ranked antioxidants. Antioxidants inhibit the oxidation of other molecules and reduce oxidative stress, the second dimension of SOWING. Berries are powerful antioxidants because berries are rich in polyphenols and contain a moderate amount of vitamin C, among many other micronutrients. Vitamin C, or ascorbic acid, is a well-known antioxidant and benefit the brain through all of the six dimensions of SOWING:

- It buffers the release of **stress hormones** in response to environmental challenges;

- It eliminates ROS and reduces **oxidative stress**;

- High dietary vitamin C or vitamin C supplementation is associated with better **work performance**, including better memory and higher capacity to pay attention and calculate. Vitamin C also protects against age-related cognitive decline;

- High intake of vitamin C enhances immunity, and reduces **inflammation** and infection. That vitamin C shortens the duration of common colds has been a well-known observation;

- Vitamin C is necessary for the synthesis of the neurotransmitter dopamine and adrenaline; it moderates neurotransmission and is essential for **neuron**al activities;

- Finally, vitamin C increases the **growth factor** BDNF in stressed animals.

Blueberries contain more polyphenols than strawberries, thus in the study introduced at the beginning of this chapter, the cognitive-enhancing effect of one or more servings of blueberries per week was bigger than that of two or more servings of strawberries per week. As good sources of polyphenols and vitamin C, berries have been attracting more attention recently.

Grapes and tomatoes are also berries

According to the Merriam-Webster dictionary, berry is "a simple fruit with a pulpy or fleshy pericarp," which includes many fruits not commonly known as berries. Examples are grapes, tomatoes (which are considered vegetables in cooking), kiwifruits, avocados, bananas, and so on. In the medical study of berries, grapes and tomatoes are often considered berries, for example, the study with a mixed berry beverage conducted at Lund University. Besides polyphenols and vitamin C, tomatoes also contain much carotenoids (mainly lycopene). As carotenoids are antioxidants and anti-inflammatory, tomatoes should have much potential to benefit the brain. But whereas there is abundant evidence that consuming tomato or tomato juice decreases the risk of chronic diseases such as cardiovascular disease and cancer, research on its cognitive-enhancing and neuroprotective effect is still scarce.

Another berry, kiwifruit is rich in polyphenols and vitamin C and contains moderate vitamin E (another antioxidant) and melatonin, a hormone modulating circadian rhythm and sleep. Rather than the cognitive-enhancing effect, kiwifruits have been investigated for their sleep-promoting effect (see Chapter 15).

Given their nutritional value and as one important family of fruit and vegetable, it is preferable to eat berries every day (see Chapter 9).

Chapter 6. Olives, for Peace and (Cognitive) Power

When I grew up in Italy in the 1950s, it was still very agricultural. Food was very important; produce was very important. Everyone made their own olive oil.

— Isabella Rossellini

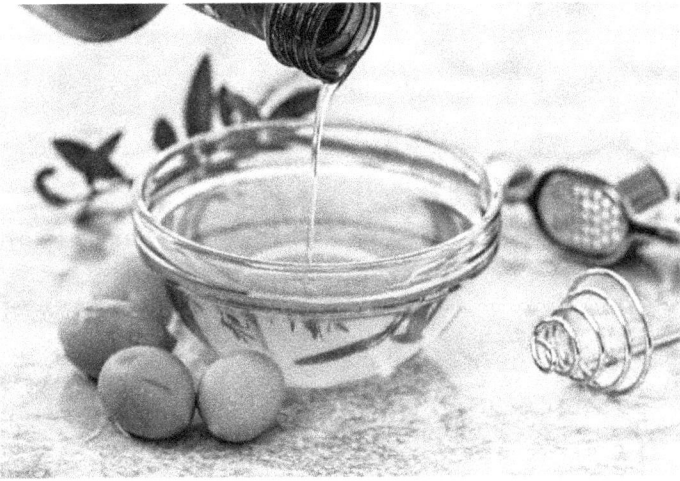

As the legend says, Zeus held a competition between Athena and Poseidon. Whoever made the most useful invention would get possession of the city. Poseidon thrust his pole weapon, a trident, into the rocky hill Acropolis. Athena planted the first olive tree. Athena's invention, useful for food, medicine, light, and heat, won. Therefore, Athens was named after her. The olive branch has become a symbol of peace and victory, while olives and olive oil are an indispensable part of the diet of those living in Athens and countries bordering the Mediterranean Sea (i.e., the Mediterranean diet, see Chapter 10).

Olives are rich in polyphenols and MUFA

Green olives contain less polyphenols than green tea and blueberry, but more than dark chocolate, cocoa, and red wine. Furthermore, olive oil is one of the major sources of monounsaturated fatty acids (MUFA) as 100 g olive oil contains 73 g MUFA (mainly oleic acid). Although olive oil also contains high amounts of saturated fat or saturated fatty acids (SFA)—the bad fat, this is not a problem here as the MUFA to SFA ratio is high and the overall health effect is positive.

MUFA, a good fat

In the current scientific literature, MUFA has been shown to positively affect four of the six dimensions of SOWING.

- MUFA reduces **oxidative stress**. MUFA possesses an antioxidant effect. It increases the resistance of low-density lipoprotein to oxidation;

- MUFA enhances work performance. **High levels of MUFA** have been shown to improve cognitive performance including the ability to pay attention, orient, and memorize. Higher MUFA to SFA ratio has been associated with slower cognitive decline;

- MUFA also reduces **inflammation**. MUFA reduces the level of and also inhibits the activity of pro-inflammatory cytokines;

- Neuroimaging research shows that MUFA enhances the **neuron**al network—the dorsal attention network—that supports general intelligence.

- In short, MUFA and polyphenols make olives powerful antioxidants and anti-inflammatory agents.

Olive oil enhances cognitive functions

The French *Three-City Study* followed the dietary habits and cognitive performance of almost 7,000 elderly adults living in Bordeaux, Montpellier, and Dijon for four years. Compared to those who never used olive oil, those who used olive oil for both cooking and dressing were at a 15% reduced risk of cognitive decline in verbal fluency and 17% reduced risk of cognitive decline in visual memory. Cooking and dressing provide two means of using olive oil, which increases the total consumption. The more total consumption, the greater the cognitive benefits.

In line with this, in a survey of almost 450 Spanish elderly individuals, the total daily consumption of olive oil was associated with the ability to memorize word lists accurately. Thus, the more total consumption, the more accurate immediate memory of word lists. Understandably, more consumption of higher quality olive oil brings greater benefits. In this study, higher use of virgin olive oil (see below), in particular, was associated with more accurate short-term memory that lasted longer than immediate memory.

Extra virgin olive oil is preferred

Among olive oils, plain olive oil is highly processed and purified using chemicals and heat. This process reduces the amount of polyphenols and produces an oil that is lighter in color and flavor. Virgin olive oil is extracted mechanically by physical pressure, without chemical extractions. Virgin olive oil with a favorable flavor is called extra virgin olive oil. Extra virgin olive oil has the deepest color and contains the greatest amount of polyphenols. A daily 25–50 ml of extra virgin olive oil is typically included in the Mediterranean diet and is known to promote good health. We mentioned that the more total consumption of olive oil, the better. But beyond daily 25–50 ml, how much more should we consume?

The randomized controlled trial PREDIMED (*Prevención con Dieta Mediterránea,* or *Primary Prevention of Cardiovascular Disease with a Mediterranean Diet*) conducted by Spanish scientists answers our question. Over 400 cognitively healthy elderly individuals from Barcelona were asked to join one of three interventions lasting six years:

- A control diet emphasizing low-fat

- An extra virgin olive oil-emphasized Mediterranean diet (for details about the Mediterranean diet, see Chapter 10), including a weekly supplementation of 1 L extra virgin olive oil

- A nuts-emphasized Mediterranean diet, including a daily supplementation of 30 g mixed nuts (15 g walnuts, 7.5 g hazelnuts, and 7.5 g almonds)

It was found that, across the six years, individuals with the control diet showed a reduction in both memory—as evaluated by immediate and delayed recall of word lists—and cognitive processing—including attention, cognitive flexibility, and working memory. Individuals with the extra virgin olive oil-emphasized Mediterranean diet showed favorable improvement on memory tests, while those with the nuts-emphasized Mediterranean diet showed favorable improvement on cognitive processing tests. It suggests that extra virgin olive oil and nuts have special benefits.

About our earlier question, weekly consumption of 1 L extra virgin olive oil or daily 140 ml (about 5 oz) is safe and beneficial, although in day-to-day life we are unlikely to use this much.

Chapter 7. Nuts: Only Skin-deep?

After-dinner talk Across the walnuts and the wine.

— Alfred Lord Tennyson
The Miller's Daughter (1842)

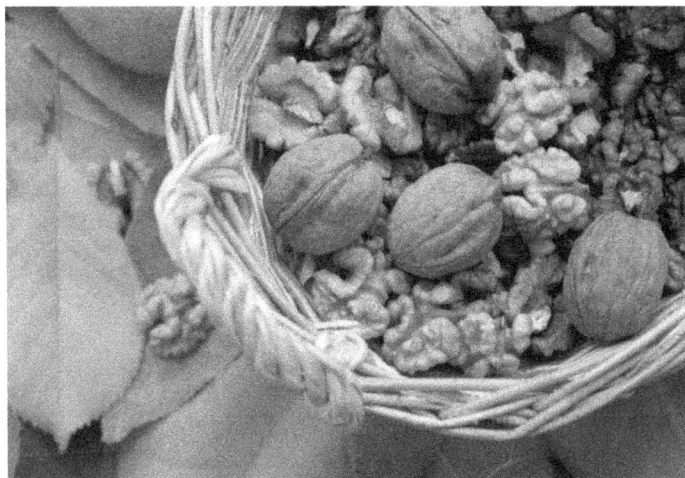

Nuts enhance cognitive functions

The benefit of nuts on cognitive functions has been well documented. In the U.S. *National Health and Nutrition Examination Survey* of adults aged 20 to 90 years, compared to those who did not consume any nuts, those who reported having consumed nuts (especially walnuts) scored higher on tests of story recall and digit–symbol substitution. The former test measures the ability to memorize, the latter the ability to process information.

In the *Nurses' Health Study* conducted by researchers at Harvard Medical School, nurses who consumed at least five servings of nuts per week had higher scores on global cognitive function than those who did not. One serving of nuts is 1 oz or 28 g.

Nuts are among the highest-ranked antioxidants

A nut is simply an oily seed in a hard shell that can be eaten as food. Examples are almonds, Brazil nuts, cashews, hazelnuts, macadamias, pecans, pine nuts, pistachios, and walnuts. Peanuts, although botanically legumes (a pod with multiple seeds), are also considered nuts here because they have a similar nutritional profile to nuts.

Nuts are particularly rich in polyphenols, including flavonoids such as catechins and flavonols, and ellagitannins. Nuts also contain a substantial amount of MUFA and vitamin E, two potent antioxidants, in addition to polyunsaturated fatty acid, plant protein, other vitamins (e.g., B6), minerals, and dietary fiber. This composition makes nuts among the highest-ranked antioxidants, comparable to berries. Among nuts, walnuts have the highest level of polyphenols and antioxidant capacity.

Nuts are only skin-deep

Remarkably, in walnuts, over 90% of polyphenols are contained in the pellicles or soft skins. In other nuts such as almonds, hazelnuts, and peanuts, more than half of polyphenols are contained in the soft skins. This is because, as we have mentioned, polyphenols are produced by plants as defense mechanisms against environmental challenges such as pathogen attacks; they have to be located on the outer side to protect the core. In addition, the outer hard shell also has a protective effect, although we do not eat this part. Nuts stored with the outer hard shell contain more polyphenols than the same nuts stored without it.

Nuts are calories dense, yet do not cause weight gain

Nuts are calories dense. Yet, epidemiological studies and clinical trials suggest that regular consumption of nuts is not associated with weight gain, and may even contribute to weight loss.

In a Spanish study of almost 9,000 college students, across the 28-month study period, compared to those who rarely consumed nuts, those who frequently consumed nuts had on average 0.42 kg less weight gain. Meanwhile, several interventional studies found that daily consumption of 30 g mixed nuts or walnuts for 3–12 months did not cause weight gain. This has been attributed to the satiating effect of nuts.

Nuts contain substantial dietary fiber, typically 6–10 g per 100 g. Some dietary fibers (known as soluble fibers) can be degraded in the colon by bacteria through the process of fermentation. This process produces short-chain fatty acids (SCFA) that enhance satiety, or make us feel full. Different from other calories dense foods, consuming food rich in dietary fibers such as nuts, whole grains (see Chapter 10), fruits, and vegetables (particularly legumes, Chapter 9) causes satiating, and helps reduce subsequent food intake thus prevents overeating. Meanwhile, SCFA has anti-**inflammatory** effects and increases the **growth factor** BDNF. Thus, high intake of dietary fiber has been found to aid weight control, reduce the risk of chronic diseases, prevent infection, and improve cognitive functions (**work performance**).

Daily 30–60 g of nuts are recommended

Research suggests that within the recommended amount of 30 g per day, there is a dose-dependent benefit on cognitive functions. Yet, consuming over 30 g per day may have a negative effect.

Scientists at Tufts University fed rats a diet containing 0%, 2%, 6%, or 9% walnuts with skins for eight weeks. Whereas the 2% and 6% diets consistently improved performance on tests of motor skills and spatial learning, the 9% diet impaired performance. The greatest benefit was at the 6% amount, which equals approximately daily 1 oz or 28 g of walnuts for humans. This amount has also demonstrated its health-promoting effects in regards to chronic diseases such as cardiovascular disease, diabetes, and cancer.

Nevertheless, researchers at Andrews University reported that, in young adults between 18–25 years old, 60 g walnuts per day for eight weeks improved performance on an inferential verbal reasoning task. The task involved the recognition of assumption, deduction, interpretation, and evaluation of verbal arguments and measured critical thinking ability. It suggests that in humans the threshold for the negative effect of nuts is higher than that in rats.

Then why does overconsumption of nuts impair cognitive performance? There are two likely reasons. First, nuts are often salted. Overconsumption of salt is harmful (see Chapter 11). Second, nuts contain much omega-6 polyunsaturated fatty acid (PUFA).

PUFA and its two families: omega-3 versus omega-6

PUFA has two families, omega-3 and omega-6. Omega-3 PUFA includes the plant omega-3 α-linolenic acid (ALA), and the animal omega-3 docosahexaenoic acid (DHA) and eicosapentaenoic acid (EPA). The plant omega-3 ALA is contained in nuts (particularly walnuts), seeds, and plant oils (such as soybean oil). The animal omega-3 DHA and EPA are primarily found in marine foods such as fish, krill, and algae.

Approximately 50–60% of the dry adult brain weight is fatty acids, of which a large proportion is DHA. DHA is an essential component of neuronal cell membranes, including those at synaptic terminals, mitochondria, and endoplasmic reticulum. Notably, omega-3 PUFA has been found to benefit the brain through all of the six dimensions of SOWING.

- It attenuates the stress response including the release of **stress hormones** in the face of environmental challenges;

- It reduces **oxidative stress** by inhibiting the production of ROS;

- It improves **work performance**: omega-3 PUFA supplements enhance memory and cognitive functions;

- It reduces **inflammation** by reducing the production of pro-inflammatory cytokines and increasing the level of adiponectin, an anti-inflammatory factor;

- It is essential for the production of **neurons**, synapses, and neurotransmitters such as noradrenaline, dopamine, and acetylcholine;

- It increases the levels of **growth factors** particularly BDNF.

Omega-6 PUFA includes linoleic acid and arachidonic acid. Dietary sources of omega-6 PUFA include plant oils such as sunflower, safflower, corn and soybean oils, nuts, and seeds. Importantly, whereas omega-3 PUFA is anti-inflammatory and reduces oxidative stress, omega-6 PUFA is pro-inflammatory and increases oxidative stress.

Furthermore, omega-6 PUFA competes for the same desaturase enzymes in the biosynthetic pathways to omega-3 PUFA. Therefore, high intake of omega-6 PUFA results in a low omega-3 PUFA status. A high ratio of omega-6: omega-3 impairs cognitive performance and increases the risk of cognitive decline and dementia.

A target ratio of 1–2:1 of omega-6: omega-3 is preferred

Whereas the ratio of omega-6: omega-3 in the western diet is estimated to be 10–20:1, a target of 1–2:1 is preferred. Therefore, it is recommended that when you eat foods rich in omega-6 PUFA, you also consume foods and/or supplements rich in omega-3 PUFA.

Walnuts have the highest level of plant omega-3 ALA among all edible plants. Yet, in walnuts, the amount of omega-3 compared to omega-6 (mainly linoleic acid) is still low, with a ratio of omega-6: omega-3 at about 5:1. In almonds, the ratio is about 38:1;

in soybean oil, 7:1; olive oil, 8:1; corn oil, 56:1; sunflower oil, 120:1.

Worse, although the plant omega-3 PUFA ALA can be converted to DHA and EPA in humans, the conversion rate is actually limited at about 5%. This highlights the importance of consuming DHA and EPA rich seafood.

Perhaps this explains why overconsumption of nuts, especially in the absence of seafood, impairs cognitive performance.

To conclude this chapter, nuts are excellent sources of polyphenols, MUFA, vitamin E, dietary fiber, and other nutrients. Daily 30–60 g of nuts is highly recommended to include as part of a healthy diet. And as such, we should also eat more omega-3 PUFA.

Chapter 8. In Search of Coldwater, Fatty Fish

I had decided that I was going to live Japanese as much as I could. That meant eating fish. I never liked fish when I was growing up, but I found out in Japan that it was a childish thing: I ate a lot of fish, and enjoyed it.

— Richard Feynman, *Surely You're Joking, Mr. Feynman!: Adventures of a Curious Character* (1985)

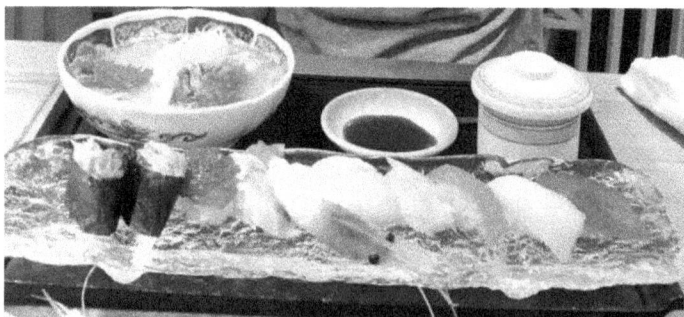

Photo: A lunch set of sushi with crab soup and soy sauce

Coldwater, fatty fish contains high levels of DHA and EPA

For the summer vacation of 2017, I went back to Hokkaido, where I received my doctorate's degree.

Hokkaido is a northern island of Japan northwest to the North Pacific Ocean, south to the Russian Sea of Okhotsk and northeast to the Sea of Japan. It is at the same latitude with Oregon, Ottawa, Jilin (China), and Northern Italy, but it is much snowier. Sapporo, its capital with a population of over two million, is one of the snowiest cities in the world, snowing for almost half the year.

Hokkaido is famous for its wildness and agriculture, including fishing. The cold sea surrounding Hokkaido is full of nutritious plankton, which attracts fish of excellent quality. From here forward, we use fish exchangeably with seafood, which includes salmon, tuna, trout, and shellfish such as shrimp, crab, and oysters. The fat in fish is adapted to its environment. Fish oil, primarily omega-3 PUFA DHA and EPA, is needed in large amounts to act as a membrane antifreeze in cold water and is essential for fish to survive. The colder the water, the higher quality the oil must be. Coldwater, fatty fish contains the best and richest omega-3 PUFA. Besides, fish are an excellent source of high-quality protein and contain many vitamins (A, D) and minerals (selenium, zinc, iodine, iron), which makes it an essential part of a healthy diet. As seafood is supplied in restaurants in Hokkaido on the same day after fishing, which keeps the freshness, no wonder some claim that Hokkaido has the best seafood in the world.

This time, we went to the Shakotan peninsula in Western Hokkaido, which is the sea urchin (Uni in Japanese) capital of Japan. Urchin in Shakotan is so delicious that my wife, who eats seafood frequently but hated urchin, loved urchin after trying it in Shakotan. Just like Richard Feynman, the Nobel laureate in Physics, who started to love fish after trying it in Japan.

Seafood enhances cognitive performance

Whereas the plasma concentrations of fatty acids reflect dietary intake over the last few days, the red blood cell (RBC) concentrations reflect dietary intake over the lifespan of RBC up to four months. It has been reported that people with high RBC levels of DHA and EPA have bigger brains, accompanied by better cognitive functions.

In line with this, in *The Optimal Well-Being, Development and Health for Danish Children through a Healthy New Nordic Diet School Meal Study*, after consuming a school meal including fish for three months, students had increased whole blood (including both plasma and RBC) levels of DHA and EPA and improved school performance in reading and math. Similarly, in a Swedish study of almost 4,000 adolescent boys, compared to those who ate fish only once or less per week, those who ate fish two or more times per week had higher IQ scores.

In the elderly, the benefits of fish are also robust. In the *Chicago Health and Aging Project* involving over 3,700 elderly people, compared to those who ate fish less than weekly, those who ate fish once per week had 10% slower cognitive decline, and those who ate fish twice or more per week had 13% slower cognitive decline. Consuming fish once or more per week was estimated to slow aging by 1.6 years in the *China Health and Nutrition Survey*.

Eating fish at least twice per week

Research suggests that even 10 g per day intake of fish and fish products is cognitively beneficial. This amount is about one serving (100 g or 4 oz) per 10 days or three servings per month. One serving is about the size and thickness of an adult's palm (see the figure below). This is the least amount necessary to benefit the brain.

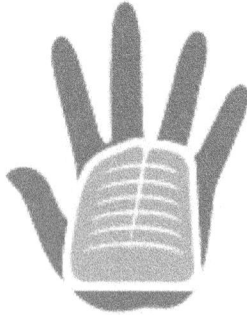

The size of one serving
of fish, about 100 g or
4 oz.

The 2015–2020 Dietary Guidelines for Americans recommends that adults should consume at least 8 oz (227 g, cooked, edible portion) of a variety of seafood per week. This is at least two servings a week. This amount is in line with the above studies that consuming at least two servings per week of fish brings a broad range of cognitive benefits. However, what amount of fish brings the greatest cognitive benefit?

In a Norwegian study of over 2,000 elderly people, the more the daily intake of fish, the better the performance on tests of cognitive functions. The greatest benefit was observed at about 75 g per day. This is about five servings per week. There is no additional cognitive benefit beyond this amount, which is likely because of "the problem" with fish.

The problem with fish

Predatory fish such as swordfish, shark, king mackerel, marlin, orange roughy, tuna, and tilefish may be contaminated with heavy, neurotoxic elements like mercury. In aquatic environments, some bacteria can methylate inorganic mercury into methylmercury, which bioaccumulates in fish. It is further biomagnified through the food chain such that predatory fish contain more mercury as they eat other mercury-containing fish; and in humans, the more fish consumption, the higher the blood levels of mercury.

Nevertheless, in general, fish consumption is associated with better cognitive functions. It suggests that if we limit seafood to those high in omega-3 PUFA but low in methylmercury, the benefits may be even greater. Examples of this kind of seafood are listed below.

A list of coldwater, fatty fish with low mercury contaminations

- Preferred choices: anchovy, Atlantic croaker, Atlantic mackerel, black sea bass, butterfish, catfish, clam, cod, crab, crawfish, flounder, haddock, hake, herring, lobster (American and spiny), mullet, Pacific chub mackerel, Pacific oysters, perch (freshwater and ocean), pickerel, plaice, Pollock, salmon, sardines, scallop, skate, shad, shrimp, smelt, sole, squid, tilapia, trout (freshwater), whitefish, whiting

- Try to avoid the following because of the high likelihood of contamination by methylmercury: swordfish, shark, king mackerel, marlin, orange roughy, tuna, and tilefish

The problem with sushi and sashimi

Cooking may reduce the concentration of omega-3 PUFA in fish. Eating raw fish, such as the Japanese style seafood, sushi, and sashimi, is a good way to retain the nutritional value. However, raw fish and undercooked fish not cooked to safe internal temperatures are at risk of contamination by microbes, including bacteria and parasites. This becomes a serious problem for individuals with low immunity, such as pregnant women, infants, children, and the elderly. As such, although fresh sushi and sashimi are nutritious and delicious, the safest choice is eating thoroughly cooked seafood.

Chapter 9. The Healthy Way (1): From "5 A Day" to "10 A Day"

The more colorful the food, the better. I try to add color to my diet, which means vegetables and fruits.

— Misty May-Treanor

Any food can be YOUR brain food

After discovering that I was writing a book on brain food, many family and friends have asked me the same question: what is the best "superfood" for the brain? Unfortunately, my answer has always been, *"Such a food doesn't exist."*

Almost all nutrients have a specific function related to one or several of the six dimensions of SOWING. Deficiencies in any nutrients can lead to poor functions of the brain. Although recently mass media frequently refer to certain foods as "superfoods," the truth is there is no single, magic food that contains all the nutrients our brain needs. Overconsumption of one food almost unavoidably causes a lack of other essential nutrients, as the amount of food we eat every day has its upper limit. Any food can be your brain food if your consumption of that food (or nutrients in that food) has been insufficient.

For instance, due to developmental need and menstruation, children and women are at high risk of iron deficiency. In these populations, consumption of iron-rich foods or iron supplements has been found to improve memory and intellectual ability. This is because iron is necessary not only in synthesizing hemoglobin for carrying oxygen, but also for forming enzymes that catalyze many processes including the biosynthesis of hormones, synapses, and neurotransmission. Lack of iron compromises the normal metabolism of the brain and its functioning. You may be interested to know that iron-rich animal foods include lean red meat such as beef and lamb, and seafood such as sardines, perch, and oysters. Iron-rich plant foods include dark green leafy vegetables (e.g., spinach and broccoli), legumes (e.g., beans, soybeans, and peas), tofu, and iron-fortified cereals, breads, and pasta.

But until causing serious, observable conditions, we seldom notice what nutrients we are lacking and when we do, it is often already too late as the damage has been done to the brain. In many cases, brain damage may be reversible, but why risk it? The best strategy is to eat a healthy, well-balanced diet that contains all the essential nutrients we need.

Patterns are all that matter: the healthy way

In real life, except for snacks, we seldom eat one food at a time. Rather, we consume a variety of foods at each meal. We have appetizers, main dishes, desserts, and beverages. Would you believe that overall food pattern matters? Emphasizing one food may bring certain health benefits, but no matter what the food, alone it cannot supply all the nutrients our body and brain need. Therefore, optimizing overall food pattern or diet quality is the most beneficial for the brain (and for overall health). The cumulative effects of multiple healthy food items will no doubt surpass individual or a few food items and result in an overall larger health benefit.

Although it is only in the past two decades that the scientific community utilized this food pattern approach, the findings have been fruitful. Research consistently shows that high-quality diets—healthy, well-balanced diets with an ideal combination of all the vital nutrients—benefit the brain in regards to all of the six dimensions of SOWING.

In students, after adjusting many confounding factors such as socioeconomic status, those with better diet quality are more likely to score high in school, show strong language and math ability, and successfully graduate.

At the workplace, those attending educational programs aimed at improving diet quality and health behaviors are more productive and are absent from work less because of illness or disability.

In the elderly, those with better diet quality are more likely to possess high cognitive abilities and less likely to show cognitive decline and develop dementia.

What, then, is a healthy, well-balanced diet?

Looking through hundreds of scientific reports, the healthy, well-balanced diets are any diets high in vegetables, fruits, and fish. These three food groups provide most, if not all, essential nutrients we need. Vegetables and fruits are rich in micronutrients, minerals, dietary fiber, and polyphenols. Fish is rich in omega-3 PUFA, protein, and vitamin D.

We have seen the cognitive-enhancing effect of fish. Below, we'll introduce a food policy called "5 A Day" on vegetables and fruits, and in the next chapter, we'll introduce the popular and frequently studied Mediterranean diet.

Vegetables and fruits: "5 A Day"

"5 A Day" is a public health slogan initiated by the World Health Organization (WHO) since 1990. To prevent chronic diseases such as cardiovascular disease, diabetes, and cancer, WHO recommends at least 400 g of fruits and vegetables daily. As one portion is defined as 80 g, this is about 5 portions.

To achieve the greatest health benefit, fruits and vegetables should include a variety of food items from different subgroups as each contain different combinations of nutrients. Fruits are good sources of vitamin C, potassium, and dietary fiber. Vegetables in the dark green subgroup provide the most vitamin K, the red and orange subgroup the most vitamin A, legumes subgroup the most dietary fiber, starchy subgroup the most potassium, and the other subgroup contain many nutrients in varying amounts. Examples of vegetables from these subgroups are:

- Dark green: dark green leafy vegetables (spinach, kale, turnip), broccoli

- Red and orange: tomatoes, red peppers, carrots, sweet potatoes, winter squash, and pumpkin

- Legumes (beans and peas): kidney beans, white beans, black beans, lentils, chickpeas, pinto beans, split peas, and edamame (green soybeans)

- Starchy: white potatoes, corn, green peas, green lima beans, plantains, and cassava

- Other: mushrooms, iceberg lettuce, green beans, onions, cucumbers, cabbage, celery, zucchini, and green peppers

To help you form an image of how 5 A Day looks like, below are several vegetables and fruits equivalent to one portion. In the case of vegetables, one portion can be:

- 1 medium tomato (tomato is a vegetable)

- 1 medium onion

- 1 green or red pepper

- 1 cereal bowl spinach

- 1 cucumber about 4 cm long

- 1 ear of corn

- 2 spears of broccoli

- 2 medium carrots

- 3 heaped tablespoons of beans or peas

- 5 spears of asparagus

For fruits, one portion can be:

- Half an avocado

- Half a grapefruit

- 1 medium apple

- 1 medium banana

- 1 medium orange

- 1 medium peach

- 1 medium pear

- 2 medium plums

- 2 kiwifruits

- 4 heaped tablespoons of blueberries

- 8 strawberries

- 9–10 blackberries

- 14 cherries

- 14 grapes

So 5 A Day can be represented by:

5 A Day

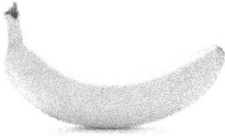
1 banana

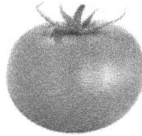
1 tomato

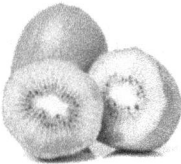
2 kiwi fruits

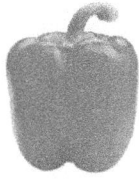
1 red pepper

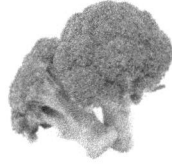
2 broccoli spears

Vegetables can be consumed fresh, frozen, canned, and as 100% vegetable juices. Fruits can be consumed fresh, frozen, canned, dried, and as 100% fruit juices. One portion of dried fruit is around 30 g or 1 oz. One portion of vegetable and fruit juice is about 150 ml or 5 oz.

High intake of vegetables and fruits not only prevents various chronic diseases and reduces mortality, but also enhances cognitive functions and buffers cognitive decline. In a Brazilian study of over 1,800 elderly people, adherence to "5 A Day" was associated with a 47% decreased risk of cognitive impairment.

From "5 A Day" to "10 A Day"

More recent research suggests that the optimum amount of vegetables and fruits may be more than five portions. A meta-analysis of 95 studies involving over two million subjects was conducted by researchers at Imperial College London and published in February 2017. The meta-analysis found a dose-dependent benefit of fruits and vegetables on mortality from all causes including cardiovascular disease, stroke, cancer, and so on. The optimum intake of fruits and vegetables is 800 g or 10 portions per day, which reduces the risk of mortality by 31%. 10 A Day can be represented by:

10 A Day

1 banana

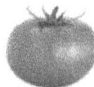
1 tomato

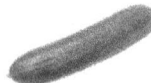
1 cucumber

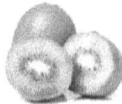
2 kiwi fruits

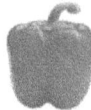
1 red pepper

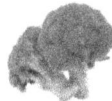
2 broccoli spears

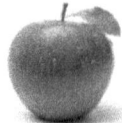
1 apple

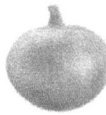
1 onion

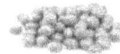
3 spoons of peas

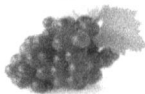
14 grapes

"10 A Day" is scientifically good, but it is rather challenging for most people to achieve. In the U.S., it is estimated that over 75% of people eat less than 5 portions of fruits and vegetables per day. Personally, after much effort, my habit now is 7–8 portions a day: one vegetable and one fruit at breakfast, two vegetables at lunch, sometimes one fruit as a snack in the afternoon, two vegetables at dinner, and one fruit as a snack in the evening.

Chapter 10. The Healthy Way (2): The Mediterranean Diet

The Mediterranean diet isn't a diet, it's a lifestyle.

— Kenton & Jane at Lemon & Olives

A report published in the journal *Lancet* in 1981 was a milestone in the field of nutritional science and public health. This report was from a 10-year follow-up study of CHD in seven developed countries, including the U.S., Finland, the Netherlands, Italy, Greece, the former Yugoslavia, and Japan. It is also known as the *Seven Countries Study*. Among the over 12,000 subjects aged 40–59 years, surprisingly, compared to the other countries, the mortality rate for CHD was about tenfold lower in the two Mediterranean countries of Italy and Greece. This low mortality rate was believed to be the result of the healthier diet in the Mediterranean area. Since then, the Mediterranean diet has received increasing attention.

The Mediterranean diet dissected

By definition, the Mediterranean diet is the traditional dietary pattern of people in countries bordering the Mediterranean Sea, notably Greece, Italy, France, Spain,

Egypt, Libya, and Algeria. The composition of the Mediterranean diet is seen in the Mediterranean Diet Pyramid, as shown in the figure below.

At the base of the pyramid are the core foods eaten at almost every meal, namely plant foods including vegetables, fruits, nuts, whole grains, olive oils, and spices (see Chapter 13). Water and wine (for those who drink alcohol) are the main beverages.

Moving upward is seafood, which is eaten at least twice a week.

Moving further up are foods eaten on a daily to weekly basis, including eggs, poultry, and dairy products (yogurt and traditional cheese).

At the top of the pyramid are foods consumed less frequently, such as red meat and processed meat products. These are typically eaten no more than a few times a month.

As you can see, this food pattern contains most of the individual food items known to promote health and enhance cognitive functions. Vegetables and fruits provide most of the micronutrients, minerals, polyphenols and dietary fiber. Fish provides abundant animal omega-3 DHA and EPA, protein and vitamin D.

Nuts and olive oil contain high levels of MUFA and considerable polyphenols. Another source of polyphenols, wine, is consumed moderately. Also, whole grains rather than refined grains are the main sources of carbohydrates.

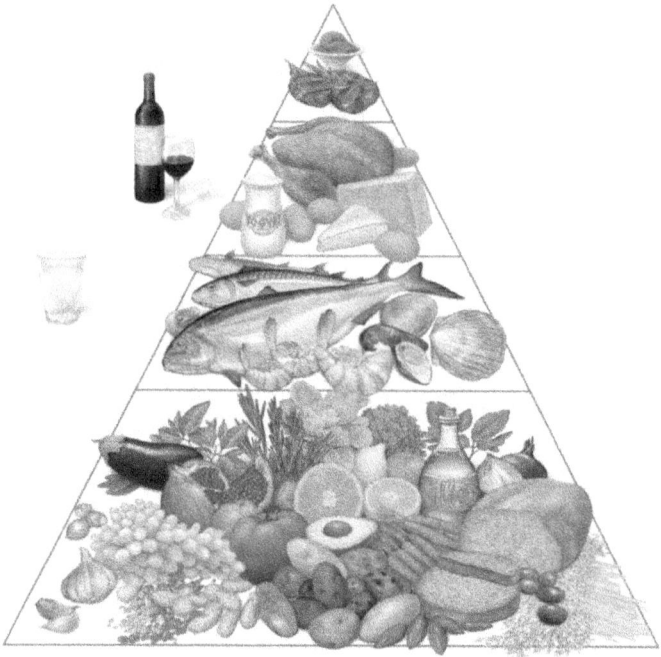

The Mediterranean Diet Pyramid (adapted). *Copyright 2009 Oldways Preservation and Exchange Trust. This pyramid was created by the Oldways Preservation and Exchange Trust, a nonprofit food and nutrition education organization, in collaboration with WHO and Harvard School of Public Health.*

Whole grains are healthier than refined ones

Refined grains are milled, a process that strips out both the bran and germ to give them a finer texture and longer shelf life, retaining only endosperm. The refining process also removes many nutrients, including dietary fiber and minerals. Refined grains include white flour, white rice, white bread and degermed cornflower. Many breads, cereals, crackers, desserts, and pastries are made with refined grains.

In contrast, whole grains haven't had their bran and germ removed by milling; therefore, all of the nutrients remain intact. Whole grains are excellent sources of dietary fiber, selenium, potassium, and magnesium. Whole grains are either single foods, such as brown rice and popcorn, or ingredients in products, such as buckwheat in pancakes or whole wheat in bread. Compared to refined grains, whole grains raise the blood level of glucose to a lower extent, which is healthier (see next chapter).

One of the healthiest diets

The Mediterranean diet is one of the healthiest diets. Dozens of observational and experimental studies have shown that stricter adherence to the Mediterranean diet is reliably related with preferable effects on the six dimensions of SOWING (stress hormones, oxidative stress, work performance, inflammation, neurons, and growth factors). In a study of 674 elderly people living in Manhattan, New York, compared to those with low adherence to the Mediterranean diet, those with high adherence had an overall bigger brain, indicating a more powerful and less atrophied brain. This effect was equivalent to about five years of aging.

The evidence strongly indicates that the Mediterranean diet contributes to a more efficient and healthy brain. This is true whether the research is conducted within the Mediterranean area or not.

Research within the Mediterranean area

Within the Mediterranean area, several famous studies, including the *Three-City Study* and the *Supplementation with Vitamins and Mineral Antioxidants* (SU.VI.MAX) Study in France, the *Nutritional aspect of the Spanish prospective cohort* (SUN project) in Spain, and the *European Prospective Investigation into Cancer and Nutrition* (EPIC) study in Greece consistently observed a positive association between high adherence to the Mediterranean diet and better cognitive functions.

In the EPIC study in the greater Athens area of Greece, higher adherence to the Mediterranean diet was associated with reduced cognitive decline in elderly people across a 7-year period. Subjects were categorized into three levels of adherence based on their diet patterns. Compared to those with low adherence, medium and high adherence was associated with a 25% and 54% lower risk of mild cognitive decline, and a 28% and 66% lower risk of substantial cognitive decline.

Research outside the Mediterranean area

Outside the Mediterranean area, research conducted in the U.S., China, and Australia has provided robust support to the cognitive benefit of the Mediterranean diet. In the *Chicago Health and Aging Project* (CHAP), the *Reasons for Geographic and Racial Differences in Stroke* (REGARDS) Study, and the *China Health and Nutrition Survey*, higher adherence to the diet was associated with slower rates of cognitive decline and a lower risk of cognitive impairment across a 4–8 year period.

As estimated by the *Chicago-based Mediterranean-dietary approach to systolic hypertension diet Intervention for Neurodegenerative Delay* (MIND) study, compared to those who had the Mediterranean diet scores in the lowest tertile (one third), those in the top tertile had cognitive functions equivalent to 7.5 years younger.

"The way not taken" is not necessarily bad: the good, the bad, and the ugly

In the Mediterranean diet, red meat and processed meat products are consumed in low amounts, no more than a few times a month. Eggs, poultry, and dairy products (yogurt and traditional cheese) are consumed in low to moderate amounts. However, these less frequently consumed foods are not necessarily bad.

A low intake of red meats such as beef, pork, lamb, veal, and goat, has frequently been associated with healthy diet patterns, which makes red meats look ugly. However, lean forms of red meat (and poultry, such as chicken, turkey, duck, geese, and guineas) provide important sources of protein, vitamins (B) and minerals (iron, zinc). Two recent surveys found that high intake of meat, particularly lean red meat, was associated with a lower risk of dementia and larger entorhinal cortical thickness. The entorhinal cortex provides the main input to the hippocampus and plays important roles in memory and navigation.

Eggs contain a relatively high level of cholesterol, which makes them look ugly. However, the effect of eggs on blood cholesterol and cardiovascular risks is relatively small compared to other truly bad foods (see below). Furthermore, eggs provide many nutrients including protein, vitamins (B), minerals (iron, zinc), choline, and bioactive compounds such as phosvitin. Choline is the precursor for the **neurotransmitter** acetylcholine and protects against **oxidative stress** and **inflammation**. In a recent Chinese survey of elderly people, high daily intake of eggs was associated with a lower risk of mild cognitive impairment, which provided the first evidence that eggs enhance **work performance**. Thus, eggs and lean red meats are actually good brain foods.

Dairy may also seem ugly due to its high saturated fat component. However, fat-free or low-fat forms of dairy promote good health (see Chapter 12).

Last, highly processed meat and meat products such as bacon, ham, lunchmeats, hot dogs, sausages, and smoked meat, and sweets are the truly bad guys, which we will introduce as part of the unhealthy diet pattern in the next chapter.

Chapter 11. The Unhealthy Way: 4 Driving Forces

You can't have a healthy civilization without healthy soil. You can't have junk food and have healthy people.

— Joel Salatin

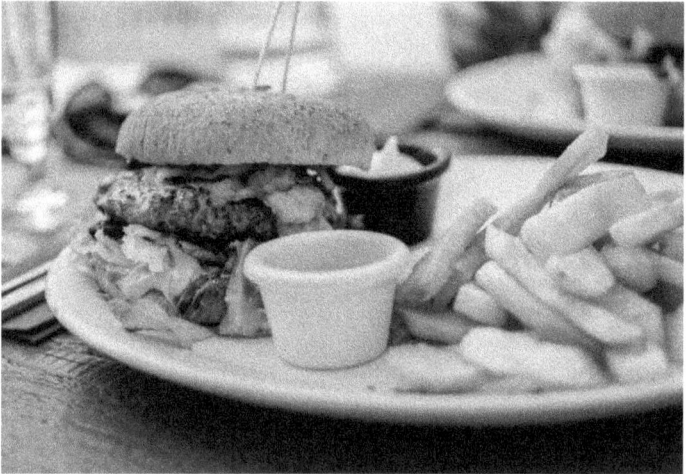

Four groups of brain junk food

Dozens of studies have indicated an unhealthy pattern that is harmful to the brain. This unhealthy pattern is characterized by high intake of any of the following foods:

- Processed meat: bacon, ham, lunchmeats, hot dogs, sausages, smoked meat

- Fried food: French fries, potato chips

- Sweets and crackers: biscuits, cakes, chocolates, cookies, pudding

- Sugar-sweetened beverages: soda/soft drinks (not sugar-free), flavored juice drinks, sports drinks, energy drinks, and coffee and tea beverages with added sugars

In children and adolescents, this pattern is associated with lower IQ, poorer linguistic, nonverbal reasoning and decision-making abilities, higher impulsivity, and worse academic achievement. In adults and the elderly, this pattern is associated with poorer executive function, memory, and linguistic abilities, and accelerated cognitive decline.

Importantly, the favorable outcomes of healthy food patterns are consistently independent of the negative outcomes of the unhealthy food pattern. It suggests that the unhealthy food pattern consists of not only a lack of healthy nutrients, but also contains toxic chemicals.

The unhealthy way dissected

Processed meat is meat transformed through salting, curing, fermentation, smoking and so on to enhance flavor and improve preservation. Compared to unprocessed meat, processed meat contains 4-fold higher levels of salt (sodium). Nutrients such as protein and iron are reduced in processed meat, while saturated fat is remained or increased.

Frying is a common cooking procedure, especially in fast food restaurants. During frying, trans fatty acids or trans fat are produced. Many sweets and crackers also contain high levels of trans fat due to high heating processing during production. Trans fat is a MUFA, but it is more like cholesterol-raising saturated fat than a MUFA. Also, cooking meat and frying at a high temperature produce carcinogenic heterocyclic amines and polycyclic aromatic hydrocarbons.

Finally, sweets, crackers, and sugar-sweetened beverages contain refined sugars and have a high glycemic index (see below). Among cakes, cheesecake, chocolate cake, and butter cake also contain high levels of saturated fat.

In conclusion, the unhealthy diet pattern contains much saturated fat, trans fat, refined sugars, and salt. These four driving forces increase the risk of chronic diseases and are harmful to the brain.

Driving force No.1: saturated fat

Ample research has been conducted on the detrimental effects of saturated fat. A diet rich in saturated fat is harmful to the brain through all of the six dimensions of SOWING.

- It changes the receptor expression of the **stress hormone** cortisol and prolongs stress response;

- It increases **oxidative stress** and oxidative damage to the brain;

- It impairs **work performance**, reduces cognitive abilities including executive function, spatial learning, and linguistic abilities, accelerates cognitive decline, and increases the risk of dementia;

- It increases **inflammation** by increasing the release of pro-inflammatory cytokines;

- It damages the **neuron**al network, reduces the production of neurons, alters the gene expression of dopamine (a neurotransmitter involved in working memory, motivation, and reward learning) and opioid (involved in reward processing), reduces serotonin (a neurotransmitter involved in stress and emotion regulation) neurotransmission.

- It reduces the level of **growth factors**, particularly BDNF in the hippocampus.

Driving force No.2: trans fat

Available evidence indicates that trans fat is more harmful than saturated fat. The cardiovascular risk of trans fat is estimated to be twice that of saturated fat. Some researchers even consider trans fat as similarly harmful to smoking, lead paint, or mercury. Within the context of SOWING, trans fat induces **oxidative stress**, and has a more severe pro-**inflammatory** effect than saturated fat. It impairs **work performance**. As shown by the *Nurses' Health Study*, compared to those with trans fat intake at the lowest tertile, those at the highest tertile on average had cognitive decline about seven years faster. In other words, if we replace trans fat with more healthy food in these subjects, we should be able to delay their cognitive aging by seven years.

Driving force No.3: refined sugars

Sweets, crackers and sugar-sweetened beverages contain high amounts of refined sugars. Refined sugars have a high glycemic index (GI). GI measures how a carbohydrate-containing food raises blood glucose. Thus, refined sugars rapidly increase blood glucose levels. When consumed in large amounts, refined sugars increase **oxidative stress** and pro-**inflammatory** cytokines. Although acutely risen blood glucose levels may bring some short-term improvement in cognitive functions, in the long-run, refined sugars alter the function of insulin receptors in the brain and cause cognitive impairment, that is, impairment in **work performance**. With sugar-sweetened beverages, as estimated by one study of over 1,600 middle school students, for each additional item consumed, the risk of hyperactivity/inattention symptoms (indicating reduced cognitive control) increased by 14%.

Refined sugars will not keep your blood sugar levels steady. That is why you will be hungry again soon. Due to excessive caloric intake, people who consume high amounts of refined sugars are more likely to become overweight and obese, which may develop into metabolic syndrome, diabetes, and/or cardiovascular disease.

Driving force No.4: salt

A high salt diet is a well-known risk factor for hypertension and cardiovascular disease. Recently it has also been shown that high salt intake impairs **work performance**. High salt intake reduces cognitive functions and is associated with accelerated cognitive decline. Two mechanisms have been proposed. First, animal experiments suggest that a high salt diet enhances **oxidative stress** in the hippocampus, which impairs spatial memory. Second, high salt intake increases blood pressure, which eventually alters brain blood supply, causes **neuron**al damage, and induces **inflammation** in the brain. As a result, cognitive impairment occurs.

The unhealthy way has many faces

We have to be very wary of the unhealthy diet pattern as it occurs in many faces and may deceive us. Fried fish, fish eaten with lots of soy sauce, salad with mayonnaise dressing (which contain much saturated fat), sugared tea and cocoa, and salted nuts, all contain healthy food items. But the unhealthy components make them potentially harmful. More importantly, foods in the unhealthy pattern are often highly tasty and induce positive emotions. Many of them can comfort people when people are stressed. Therefore, these foods are usually referred to as "comfort food." But they are actually brain junk foods (see Chapter 14). The take home message is that it is essential to enhance your ability to identify the four unhealthy driving forces in your daily diet.

Chapter 12. The Case for Dairy

I had an alarm, I had nerve gas, I had a yogurt. What more could anyone want?

— Janet Evanovich, *One For The Money: A Stephanie Plum Novel* (1999)

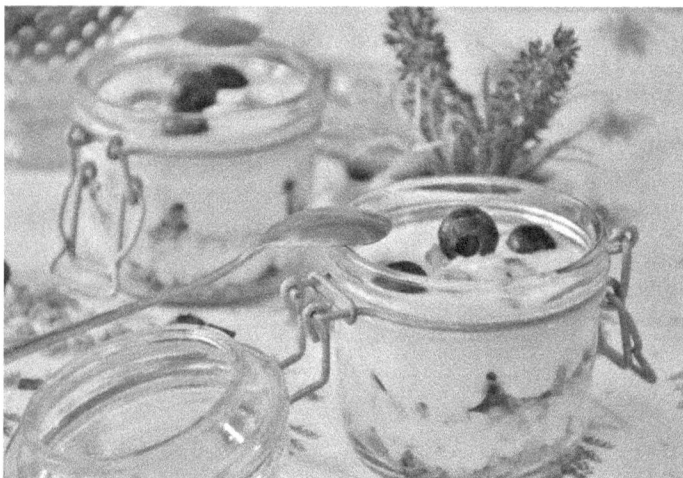

Perhaps dairy is most well-known for its health-promoting effect on bones. Milk, yogurt, cheese and milk products provide a rich source of minerals (calcium, potassium, magnesium, zinc), vitamins (D, A, B12, riboflavin), and high-quality protein. Fortified soy beverages or soymilk fortified with calcium, vitamin A, and D are also considered dairy because of their similarity in nutritional composition and use in meals.

Fat-free or low-fat dairy reliably enhances cognitive functions

Three trends have arisen from recent research. First, although there exists insignificant even negative findings, the evidence overall supports the view that dairy improves cognitive functions and prevents cognitive decline. In a survey of over 600 Korean high school students, more frequent milk consumption was associated with better academic performance in math and social science. Further analysis showed that students who consumed milk frequently had better learning and testing skills. A meta-analysis of seven studies involving over 10,000 elderly subjects was reported in 2016. It concluded that the highest milk consumption was associated with a 28% reduced risk of cognitive disorders such as Alzheimer's disease.

Second, saturated fat from dairy—for instance, in some whole fat milk, cheese, desserts, ice cream, and cream—is bad and associated with poorer cognitive functions. We have seen the harmful effects of saturated fat in Chapter 11. This may explain why research on the benefit of whole fat dairy is somewhat inconsistent.

Third, understandably, the consumption of fat-free (skim) or low-fat (1%) dairy is more beneficial than whole fat dairy. Research on the benefits of fat-free and low-fat dairy is more consistent. In a survey of almost 1,200 South Australian adults, frequent intake of low-fat dairy was associated with better cognitive and social functioning. Another experiment also conducted by Australian scientists provided further support. In this experiment, overweight subjects were randomly assigned to a high-dairy or low-dairy group. Those in the high-dairy group were instructed to consume four daily servings of low-fat dairy products including milk, yogurt, and custard. Those in the low-dairy group were instructed to consume one serving of dairy or less per day. After maintaining this diet style for six months, those who consumed four servings per day had improved working memory.

In addition, dairy intake, particularly low-fat dairy and yogurt, reduces the risk of cardiovascular disease, type 2 diabetes, hypertension, and metabolic syndrome.

Three cups of fat-free or low-fat dairy per day

The 2015–2020 Dietary Guidelines for Americans recommends three cups of fat-free or low-fat dairy per day for all adults. One cup of dairy equals one measured cup (8 oz or 237 ml) of milk, yogurt, or soymilk.

Fat-free or low-fat milk and yogurt are preferred over cheese, as the former contain less saturated fat and sodium, and more vitamin A, D, and potassium. Furthermore, avoid dairy sweetened with added sugars, such as flavored milk, yogurt, and various desserts.

Yogurt and gut microbiota

Yogurt has been consumed and used to treat diarrhea for centuries by both the layperson and the physician. Yet, it was not until the twentieth century that scientists explained its health benefit. In 1905, a Bulgarian medical student Stamen Grigorov first discovered Bacillus bulgaricus (now L. bulgaricus), a lactic acid bacteria in yogurt. Based on this finding, in 1907, the Russian scientist Yllia Metchnikoff, who would go on to receive his Nobel Prize in Physiology or Medicine a year later, suggested that the longevity of the Bulgarian peasant may be due to the bacteria in yogurt they frequent consumed. After over a century of research, it has now become evident that the bacterial strains in yogurt are health-promoting.

In the human gut (and on the skin), there are different strains of bacterial species. Some are needed to digest dietary fibers, while some produce nutrients like vitamin K. An optimal balance in the intestinal microflora is essential for health. Lactobacillus and Bifidobacterium, two strains commonly fermented in yogurt, play pivotal roles in this balance. Increasing evidence indicates that certain bacteria of these strains have many benefits in regards to inflammatory disease, obesity, and diabetes, and also promote brain health. They attenuate the release of **stress hormones**, reduce **oxidative stress**, are important for **work performance** including spatial memory and may play a role in preventing cognitive decline, reduces **inflammation**, modulates **neurotransmission**, and increase **growth factors** particularly BDNF. The pathways behind these effects are known as the brain-gut-microbiota axis (microbiota refers to the microbial population present in the human body).

In the context of these findings, many companies have developed commercial probiotics, which are believed to promote health through the actions on the brain-gut-microbiota axis. Meanwhile, Asian people have long been consuming many bacteria fermented foods based on milk (calpis sour milk), soybeans (soy sauce, soybean paste such as miso and Cheonggukjang, natto), rice (hongqu or koji, rice vinegar), and vegetables (kimchi). Several reports supporting the favorable effect of probiotics and many fermented foods on cognitive functions have been published in animals. But to my knowledge, no study has been done in humans through December 2017. Hopefully, I can update you on the benefit of these promising brain foods in humans in the second edition of this book.

Chapter 13. Spices, as Precious as Gold

But in truth, should I meet with gold or spices in great quantity, I shall remain till I collect as much as possible, and for this purpose I am proceeding solely in quest of them.

— Christopher Columbus, Friday, 19 October 1492

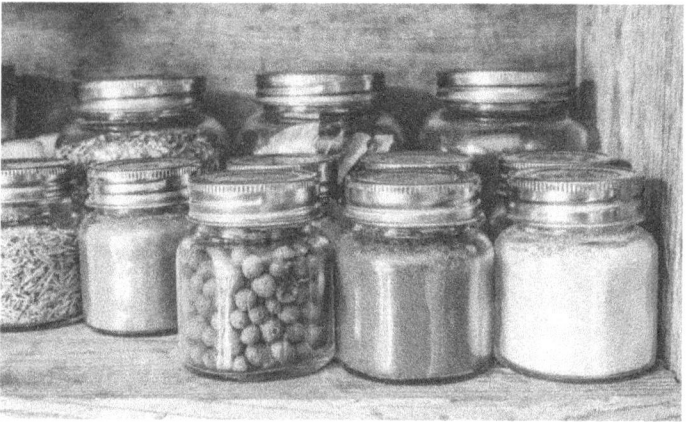

Historically, spices were as precious as gold. Many "explorers" set out their historic expeditions to find gold and spices. Spices have been used in cuisines and as medicines for thousands of years. It is a certainty that the benefit of spices extends beyond their tastes and flavors. Although consumed in only small quantities every day, the contribution of spices to human health is nevertheless of great significance.

Spices are powerful antioxidants

Research has long documented the benefits of spices in preventing and treating cardiovascular disease, cancer, infections, and neurodegenerative diseases. But it is only recently that the chemical components and biological actions of spices have been illuminated. Bio-assay studies suggested that spices (with herbs) are the highest-ranked antioxidants in all natural products. They have antioxidant contents such as polyphenols that are several folds higher than that in nuts and berries. Spices are also important brain foods, although research on spices has been primarily conducted in animals.

Garlic, ginger, and cognitive functions in animal research

Cinnamon and black pepper have just demonstrated their neuroprotective effects in animal models of Alzheimer's disease in two papers published in 2015, respectively. Garlic, ginger, and turmeric have been investigated more extensively.

Garlic is stinky for some people and it is considered rude to eat garlic before meeting important persons. As an alternative, aged garlic extract (AGE), a concentrated form of garlic and odorless, has received much attention and developed as a dietary supplement. AGE has been shown to improve memory and cognitive performance in animal models of aging and Alzheimer's disease.

Ginger is a special spice. It can inhibit the activity of acetylcholinesterase, an enzyme that breaks down the neurotransmitter acetylcholine. Thus, ginger increases the level of acetylcholine in the brain. Acetylcholine is an excitatory neurotransmitter that enhances neurotransmission and cognitive abilities. Notably, acetylcholine is decreased in patients with Alzheimer's disease and increasing acetylcholine is one of the major clinical treatment targets. Therefore, ginger has been shown to enhance cognitive abilities in normal animals and ameliorate cognitive impairment in animal models of Alzheimer's disease and memory deficits.

Turmeric and curry

Turmeric is a yellow curry spice. It is known as ''yellow ginger'' among the Chinese and a major constituent of the traditional Chinese medicine Xiaoyao-san, an antidepressant.

Curcumin is a compound isolated from turmeric and is the primary supplier of yellow pigmentation. Curcumin possesses potent anti**oxidant** and anti-

inflammatory properties. Chronic administration of curcumin in stressed animals attenuates the release of **stress hormones** and increases the level of the **growth factor** BDNF. Curcumin can cross the blood-brain barrier and directly bind to the small amyloid beta-protein oligomer to prevent amyloid beta-protein aggregation, which protects the **neuron**al network and reduces the progression of Alzheimer's disease. That is, curcumin can decrease reduction in **work performance**.

The wide use of turmeric in India is believed to contribute to the low incidence of Alzheimer's disease in the country: the prevalence of Alzheimer's disease in adults aged 70-79 years in India is over four times less than that in the U.S. In accordance with this theory, in the *Singapore National Mental Health Survey of the Elderly* of over 1,000 elderly people, compared to those who never or rarely consumed curry, those who consumed curry once a month or more often had a 49% reduced risk of cognitive impairment.

PART 2. FOOD FOR FEELINGS AND SLEEP

Chapter 14. Mood-boosting Foods

After a good dinner one can forgive anybody.

— Oscar Wilde, *A Woman of No Importance* (1893)

Humans are emotional animals. Every day we live and work with feelings and mood swings. To live a better life, we need to feel right. Even when things go wrong, we may feel negative for a while, but we can eventually achieve control and peace, and move on. This is reflected in an overall more positive and less negative mood. To achieve this emotional wellbeing, our education, psychological literacy, personality, and personal discipline come into play. But our diet is also important.

Feelings, or moods, are the output of the brain

Although the exact mechanism of how our feelings arise in our mind remains unclear (which is the subject of the field of consciousness research), it is obvious that our feelings are influenced by stress hormones, oxidative stress, inflammation, and growth factors, and are based on the neuronal network. When we feel stressed, our body releases a large amount of stress hormones. The level of oxidative stress and inflammation also increase.

These negative outcomes reduce growth factors and are harmful to neurons, neurogenesis, and neurotransmission. When the stressor is prolonged, we may eventually become burned out or depressed.

On one hand, people receiving cortisone (a precursor to the stress hormone cortisol) therapies or with conditions of high oxidative stress, inflammation, or neuronal damage such as metabolic syndrome, cardiovascular diseases, diabetes, stroke, dementia, and Parkinson's disease are more likely to develop depression. On the other hand, physical exercise, psychological therapies, and antidepressants reduce people's feelings of stress and depression by modulating neurotransmission, reducing stress hormones, oxidative stress, inflammation, and increasing growth factors.

Therefore, feelings are the output of the brain and belong to the dimension of work performance in our SOWING model.

The cognitive effect of feelings

A theme emerged from recent affective neuroscience and positive psychology is that feelings are not only our internal sensations, but also affect our cognitive abilities. Negative feelings of stress, burnout, and sadness, not only feel painful but also impair our cognitive abilities. Positive feelings such as happiness, satisfaction, and gratitude, not only feel good but also enhance our cognitive abilities.

To illustrate this point, here I borrow one example I have given in my previous book *Fitness Powered Brains*. Harvard management scientist Teresa Amabile found that company employees' moods on the previous day predicted their creative thinking and performance the next day. Positive moods on the previous day were associated with more creative ideas and higher performance, while negative moods were associated with less creative ideas and lower performance.

Keep your feelings in check

It is wise to keep your feelings in check. I have created several online tests of negative and positive feelings; get your automatic feedback here:
https://brainandlife.net/psychological-tests/

The healthy food patterns for feelings

As feelings and moods are the output of the brain, diets, which powerfully modulate the brain through the six dimensions of SOWING, can regulate feelings.

If you eat right for thoughts, you are also eating right for feelings. Foods for thought are also foods for feelings. Decades of research indicate that the overall healthy food pattern for feelings is also characterized by high intake of fruits, vegetables, and fish. This healthy pattern reduces stress hormones and the feeling of stress in response to environmental challenges.

The Mediterranean diet, which contains abundant vegetables, fruits and fish, is a well-accepted healthy food pattern for feelings. In one experiment conducted by Australian scientists, young women were randomly assigned to a diet change or control group. Only those in the diet change group were instructed to switch to a Mediterranean-style diet. Merely ten days after the diet change, these women reported increased positive feelings of vigor, alertness, and contentment, and reduced feeling of confusion. They also showed statistically significant improvement on a memory recall task. One may argue that perhaps these effects were simply because of the change and novelty factor, which rescues one out of habitual routines. But further experiments and other evidence suggest otherwise.

In a second Australian experiment, compared to those receiving a "befriending" protocol in which subjects met with research staff discussing neutral topics of interest (sport, news, music), depressed patients receiving instructions on a Mediterranean-style diet displayed more reduced symptoms of depression and a higher likelihood of remission 12 weeks later. Similarly, in a third experiment, compared to a low-fat diet change, a Mediterranean diet change combined with daily 30 g of nuts reduced the risk of depression by 22% three years later in Spanish elderly people.

These findings suggest that the Mediterranean diet—not just change in general—improves feelings. In fact, dozens of surveys have reported that the stricter the adherence to the Mediterranean diet, the more positive emotions, greater satisfaction with one's health, and fewer symptoms of depression one experiences.

The unhealthy food pattern for feelings

The unhealthy food pattern for feelings is characterized by high intake of processed meat, fried food, sweets, crackers, and sugar-sweetened beverages. It contains much saturated fat, trans fat, refined sugars, and sodium. These four unhealthy driving forces have been associated with negative feelings such as depression.

A typical food of an unhealthy diet, fast food such as hamburgers, pizza, and sausages are junk foods. That is not only because they increase the risk of obesity and chronic diseases, but also because they damage our brain and reduce our cognitive ability. Worse, they are harmful to our emotional wellbeing. This is somewhat surprising, as fast food is generally palatable, tasty, and enjoyable.

Recent research conducted by Canadian scientists suggested that fast food may actually reduce our ability to savor. To savor means to derive pleasurable feeling from everyday experiences. This may be because fast food changes the brain reward system. Animal experiments show that a diet high in saturated fat decreases the turnover of dopamine in the nucleus accumbens, one brain area of the reward system. Dopamine released in this area is associated with the anticipation and hedonic experiencing of rewards. In line with this, rats fed with a diet high in saturated fat show reduced operant responding for sucrose. This is weird in normal rats because they love sucrose; when you give them a dip of sucrose each time they press a bar, they will keep pressing it to get more sucrose. Thus, fast food attenuates our ability to savor. Eventually, fast food harms our ability to feel right. A Spanish cohort study of almost 9,000 people for over six years estimated that those with high consumption of fast food were at a 36% increased risk of developing depressive disorders.

The case against comfort food

Fast food is one example of comfort food. As the name reveals, comfort food refers to food that comforts people, such as fast food and sweets (including milk chocolate), which are characterized by high saturated fat and refined sugar. These foods are highly tasty and bring positive feelings. When stressed, many people (particularly women, as data show) turn to these foods for comfort.

Immediately after consumption, comfort food efficiently attenuates the release of stress hormones and relaxes people. This pattern of behavior is known as emotional eating, as the driving motivation and end of eating is emotional. And the end of eating indeed is emotional:

- After emotional eating, many people soon feel guilty, because they often realize the unhealthy consequences of emotional eating.

- In the long-run, emotional eating worsens people's ability to savor and increases negative feelings besides cardiovascular risks.

- Emotional eating impairs impulse control. Highly "tasty" diets high in saturated fat and refined sugar reduce one's ability for self-control, which consequently increases impulsivity and uncontrolled eating and eventually leads to overweight and obesity.

Remember this dark side of enjoyment with emotional eating, and stay away from comfort food. When stressed, use effective strategies to soothe yourself. For instance, you can exercise (see *Fitness Powered Brains*), approach nature (see *CleverLand: How Nature Nurtures*), or talk to family, friends, and medical professionals. Eating right, even in stressful situations, is the key to long-lasting happiness.

Chapter 15. Foods That Help You Sleep

One cannot think well, love well, sleep well, if one has not dined well.

— Virginia Woolf, *A Room of One's Own* (1929)

The function of sleep in a healthy brain

We spend almost one-third of our life asleep, seemingly doing nothing. Yet, sleep is a vital part of our lives. Sleep recharges us after a full day of work. Furthermore, two important neural processes occur during sleep: the consolidation of memory (the incorporation of new memory into previous knowledge) and the clearance of beta-amyloid (the metabolic trash of the brain and a driver of Alzheimer's disease). Those who suffer from sleep problems are also more likely to suffer from cognitive and emotional issues.

Are you sleeping well?

When you get a good night of sleep, you fall asleep easily in a couple of minutes after going to bed and closing your eyes. It may take you longer, but generally no longer than 30 minutes. A second feature is that you do not wake up in the middle of sleep. Even if you do, it typically occurs no more than once a night, and you can easily fall back asleep again. A third feature is that you feel refreshed in the morning after waking up. A fourth feature is that you do not have trouble staying awake during the day at work and while doing other activities.

If your sleep fails these features, you have difficulty initiating sleep (prolonged sleep latency) and maintaining sleep, and your sleep is non-restorative. In other words, you may be suffering from insomnia.

You can take a sleep quality test at https://brainandlife.net/test-sleep-quality to see if you are sleeping well. Read my blog post "Twelve Tips to Help You Get a Better Sleep" (https://brainandlife.net/2017/09/10/twelve-tips-to-help-you-get-a-better-sleep/) and the rest of this chapter carefully to improve your sleep. Refer to a doctor if necessary.

The neurobiology of sleep

We sleep at night and get up in the morning. Our bodies work best under this routine or circadian rhythm. It is controlled by a hormone called melatonin. Melatonin is secreted by the pineal gland in response to variations in the circadian cycle. The secretion is suppressed by the exposure of the retina to light and most active at night. That is, melatonin conveys information about the lightness-darkness cycle. The information is delivered to the whole body for the organization of physiological activities, such as the sleep-wake rhythms and the nocturnal core temperature. In fact, melatonin is widely used as sleeping pills to treat sleep disorders.

A diet approach towards getting a good night of sleep is scientifically sound, as melatonin is a hormone and its secretion is affected by diet: the components come from food anyway. Thus, there are at least three ways we can improve our sleep through diet.

First, consume all the nutrients necessary for the synthesis and functioning of melatonin. There is robust evidence that deficiencies in vitamins (B12, D) and minerals (magnesium, zinc) disrupt sleep. With this in consideration, the overall diet approach is preferred. Second, avoid foods that negatively affect sleep at dinner or before sleep, including those that increase arousal and/or inhibit the synthesis of melatonin. Third, eat foods that promote the synthesis of melatonin at dinner or before sleep. Combining these three ways will have the greatest benefits on sleep.

A healthy diet for thought is also a sleep diet

A healthy diet for thought is also a healthy diet for sleep, while an unhealthy diet for thought impairs sleep. Diets high in vegetables, fruits, and fish are associated with better sleep, while diets high in processed meat, fried foods, sweets and sugar-sweetened beverages are associated with sleep problems. The Mediterranean diet is again a healthy diet for sleep: those who adhere to the Mediterranean diet more strictly are more likely to have a good night of sleep and less likely to develop insomnia.

Bad foods that prevent you from a good night of sleep

There is strong evidence that intake of caffeine several hours (which varies according to individual difference) before sleep causes difficulty in falling asleep. If you regularly drink coffee, tea or other beverages containing caffeine several hours before bedtime and yet sleep well, perhaps you don't have to give up your habit. However, if you do have trouble falling asleep, you'd better make some changes. For instance, if you are a tea lover but are sensitive to caffeine, consider a low-caffeine or caffeineless tea. Low-caffeine green tea has been shown to promote sleep. Green tea is rich in polyphenols, which help reduce stress and mental fatigue, negative influencers of sleep.

Another sleep-unfriendly food is alcohol. Drinking alcohol before bedtime increases sleepiness and may help induce sleep, but it also disturbs your deep sleep and causes you to wake up in the middle of sleep. The harmful effect is obvious with heavy drinking, which causes insomnia. As we have said, women are more sensitive to alcohol. Whereas four drinks a day is heavy drinking for men, two drinks a day is heavy drinking for women.

Sleep diets: foods that promote sleep

Theoretically, food rich in melatonin, if consumed at dinner or before bedtime, promotes sleep. Examples of such food include milk, several fruits (grapes, cherries, strawberry), mushrooms, nuts (pistachio has the highest melatonin among all foods), eggs and fish. But to date, scientists have only studied four foods: milk, cherry, kiwifruit, and fish.

Sleep foods

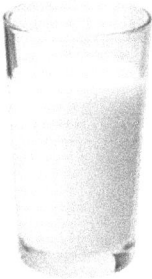
Milk

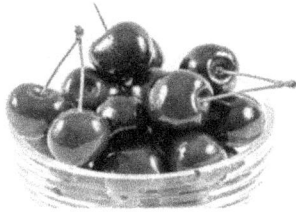
Cherries

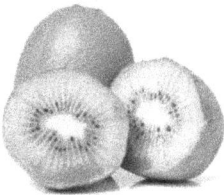
Kiwifruits

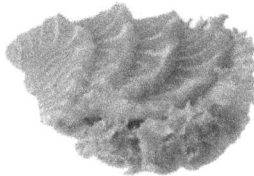
Fish

There are reports that drinking milk (e.g., 350 ml) 30–60 minutes before bedtime reduces night awakenings, although non-significant findings also exist. Perhaps the concentration of melatonin in cow milk is still relatively low. When cows are milked in darkness at nighttime, the concentration of melatonin increases substantially. This milk is called melatonin-rich nighttime milk and its sleep-promoting effect is robust. In addition, probiotic fermented milk promotes sleep. In two Japanese studies, whereas Lactobacillus helveticus fermented milk improved sleep efficiency and reduced night awakenings in elderly people, Lactobacillus casei strain Shirota fermented milk maintained the sleep quality of college students even in the face of an academic examination.

Cherry and kiwifruit are rich in melatonin. 8 oz tart cherry juice, 200 g Jerte Valley cherries, or 2 kiwifruits consumed 1–2 hours before bedtime have been found to promote sleep in adults.

Fish is rich in DHA and vitamin D, two nutrients that increase melatonin. Surveys show that regular consumption of fish is associated with better sleep quality. One experiment reported that salmon consumed three times per week promoted sleep.

PART 3. CONCLUSION

Chapter 16. We Are What We Eat

Tell me what you eat and I will tell you who you are.

— Jean Anthelme Brillat-Savarin, *The Physiology of Taste* (1825)

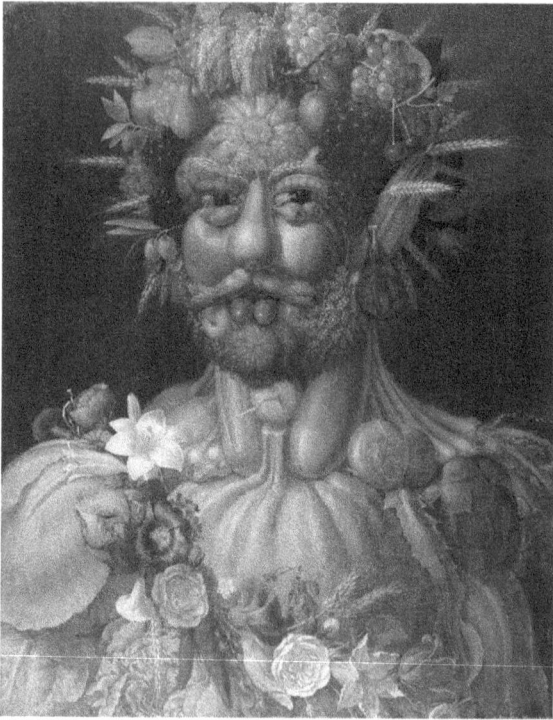

Vertumnus. A portrait by Italian painter Giuseppe Arcimboldo depicting Rudolf II, Holy Roman Emperor painted as Vertumnus, the Roman God of the seasons, c. 1590-1. Skokloster Castle, Sweden.

What we eat determines how we think, feel, and whether we can sleep soundly or not. Based on René Descartes' famous proposition "*I think, therefore I am*," saying "*we are what we eat*" is not an exaggeration. We have gone through the journey from chocolate and the Nobel Prize to a list of brain foods and junk foods. Our next task is to integrate the brain foods and eliminate or reduce the junk foods from our daily diets.

How to start your brain food revolution

Every time you eat or drink, you get an opportunity to improve.

If you drink milk at breakfast, make it skim or low-fat, or switch it up and opt for yogurt sometimes.

If you eat sandwichs, replace bacon with seafood or eggs and add more colorful vegetables.

If you use mayonnaise for salad, swap it with olive oil.

If you cook, replace palm oil with olive oil and add some spices.

If you eat bread, try to choose whole wheat bread.

If you eat white rice, try brown rice.

If you eat sausages, change to lean red meat and poultry.

If you eat meat or poultry every day, try to replace two or three meals with seafood every week.

If you eat crackers and sweets as snacks, try fruits and nuts; and if you are obsessed with chocolate, limit yourself to dark chocolate and reduce the frequency to twice or thrice a week.

If you drink soda or cola, try tea and 100% fresh vegetable or fruit juice.

If you drink sugar-sweetened milk tea, make it green tea.

If you drink spirits, limit it to one to two drinks a day, and try wine sometimes.

Use these opportunities and, eventually, you'll revolutionize your diet habit. Recall the experiment we introduced earlier. Merely ten days after switching to the Mediterranean diet, people displayed robust improvement in memory and feelings. And you too can experience that improvement.

Food versus supplement

As a rule of thumb, foods are safer and more beneficial than supplements. Food contains a variety of nutrients while supplements typically contain a single or limited nutrients. Besides, food is tastier than supplements. Whenever foods are available, choose foods; when foods are not available, use highly selected supplements.

Personalize your dietary habits

We make decisions about food several times a day. These decisions are actually the results of a complex interaction of at least four factors:

- Our beliefs about the nutritional value of a certain food, whether the belief is scientifically true or not

- Our preference towards certain foods, including physical allowance due to allergies

- Cultural and situational considerations, such as choices at parties, festivals, or on special days

- The availability of foods such as cost and local supply

Throughout this book, we have introduced a list of brain foods and junk foods, which we hope have updated your beliefs. As the next step, it is your turn to weigh your preference, the situation, availability and your updated beliefs to determine your everyday diets. But again, the final message we want to tell you is, whatever your situation, you can always improve your diet. You can always make small changes to your diet to help you think more effectively, feel more positively, and sleep more soundly. Good luck.

Postscript

At the beginning of this book, I hated chocolate. Now, I have a more balanced, scientific viewpoint of chocolate: dark chocolate is a brain food and can be consumed in moderate amounts. My wife also refreshed her point of view and realized that, to optimize her chance of receiving the phone call from the Nobel Committee in Stockholm, she has to eat a variety of brain foods.

I hope this book has helped you form a balanced, scientific view of food as well. If you want to learn more about brain foods, sign up to my newsletters at http://brainandlife.net and follow me on twitter @ChongChenBlog. I will share more research digests with you.

If you enjoyed this book, please leave a brief review on Amazon or Goodreads to let more people discover it. Thanks.

REFERENCES

Chapter 1. Introduction

Messerli, F.H. (2012) Chocolate consumption, cognitive function, and Nobel laureates. *N Engl J Med*. 367(16):1562-4.

Maurage, P., Heeren, A., & Pesenti, M. (2013). Does chocolate consumption really boost Nobel award chances? The peril of over-interpreting correlations in health studies. *The Journal of nutrition*, 143(6), 931-933.

Golomb, B. A. (2013). Lab life: Chocolate habits of Nobel prizewinners. *Nature*, 499(7459), 409-409.

Chapter 2. Chocolate, a Double-edged Sword

The health benefits of 2–3 servings of chocolate per week

Yuan, S., Li, X., Jin, Y., & Lu, J. (2017). Chocolate consumption and risk of coronary heart disease, stroke, and diabetes: A Meta-analysis of prospective studies. *Nutrients*, 9(7), 688.

Gong, F., Yao, S., Wan, J., & Gan, X. (2017). Chocolate Consumption and Risk of Heart Failure: A Meta-Analysis of Prospective Studies. *Nutrients*, 9(4), 402.

Nurk, E., Refsum, H., Drevon, C. A., Tell, G. S., Nygaard, H. A., Engedal, K., & Smith, A. D. (2009). Intake of flavonoid-rich wine, tea, and chocolate by elderly men and women is associated with better cognitive test performance. *The Journal of nutrition*, *139*(1), 120-127.

Lamuela-Raventós, R. M., Romero-Pérez, A. I., Andrés-Lacueva, C., & Tornero, A. (2005). Health effects of cocoa flavonoids. *Revista de Agaroquimica y Tecnologia de Alimentos*, *11*(3), 159-176.

Sokolov, A. N., Pavlova, M. A., Klosterhalfen, S., & Enck, P. (2013). Chocolate and the brain: neurobiological impact of cocoa flavanols on cognition and behavior. *Neuroscience & Biobehavioral Reviews*, 37(10), 2445-2453.

Williams, R. J., & Spencer, J. P. (2012). Flavonoids, cognition, and dementia: actions, mechanisms, and potential therapeutic utility for Alzheimer disease. *Free Radical Biology and Medicine*, *52*(1), 35-45.

The "sowing" power of polyphenols

Del Rio, D., Rodriguez-Mateos, A., Spencer, J. P., Tognolini, M., Borges, G., & Crozier, A. (2013). Dietary (poly) phenolics in human health: structures, bioavailability, and evidence of protective effects against chronic diseases. *Antioxidants & redox signaling*, *18*(14), 1818-1892.

Pandey, K. B., & Rizvi, S. I. (2009). Plant polyphenols as dietary antioxidants in human health and disease. *Oxidative medicine and cellular longevity*, *2*(5), 270-278.

Tangney, C. C., & Rasmussen, H. E. (2013). Polyphenols, inflammation, and cardiovascular disease. *Current atherosclerosis reports*, *15*(5), 324.

Caruana, M., Cauchi, R., & Vassallo, N. (2016). Putative role of red wine polyphenols against brain pathology in Alzheimer's and Parkinson's disease. *Frontiers in nutrition*, *3*.

Opie, L. H., & Lecour, S. (2007). The red wine hypothesis: from concepts to protective signalling molecules. *European heart journal*, *28*(14), 1683-1693.

Zhu, W. L., Shi, H. S., Wei, Y. M., Wang, S. J., Sun, C. Y., Ding, Z. B., & Lu, L. (2012). Green tea polyphenols produce antidepressant-like effects in adult mice. *Pharmacological Research*, *65*(1), 74-80.

Lee, J. B., Shin, Y. O., Min, Y. K., & Yang, H. M. (2010). The effect of Oligonol intake on cortisol and related cytokines in healthy young men. *Nutrition research and practice*, *4*(3), 203-207.

Poulose SM, Miller MG, Scott T, Shukitt-Hale B. (2017) Nutritional Factors Affecting Adult Neurogenesis and Cognitive Function. *Adv Nutr*. 8(6):804-811.

Evans, H. M., Howe, P. R., & Wong, R. H. (2017). Effects of Resveratrol on Cognitive Performance, Mood and Cerebrovascular Function in Post-Menopausal Women; A 14-Week Randomised Placebo-Controlled Intervention Trial. *Nutrients*, *9*(1), 27.

Serafini, M., Bugianesi, R., Maiani, G., Valtuena, S., De Santis, S., & Crozier, A. (2003). Plasma antioxidants from chocolate. *Nature*, *424*(6952), 1013-1013.

Dark chocolate is better than white

Fernández-Murga, L., Tarín, J. J., García-Perez, M. A., & Cano, A. (2011). The impact of chocolate on cardiovascular health. *Maturitas*, *69*(4), 312-321.

Tara Parker-Pope (2007 December) The Problem With Chocolate. Available https://well.blogs.nytimes.com/2007/12/21/the-problem-with-chocolate/ (last accessed 2017-12-04)

The problem with chocolate

Greenberg, J. A., Manson, J. E., Buijsse, B., Wang, L., Allison, M. A., Neuhouser, M. L., ... & Thomson, C. A. (2015). Chocolate-candy consumption and 3-year weight gain among postmenopausal US women. *Obesity*, 23(3), 677-683.

Light brown natural cocoa can be consumed daily

Socci, V., Tempesta, D., Desideri, G., De Gennaro, L., & Ferrara, M. (2017). Enhancing Human Cognition with Cocoa Flavonoids. *Frontiers in Nutrition*, *4*.

Katz, D. L., Doughty, K., & Ali, A. (2011). Cocoa and chocolate in human health and disease. *Antioxidants & redox signaling*, *15*(10), 2779-2811.

Sokolov, A. N., Pavlova, M. A., Klosterhalfen, S., & Enck, P. (2013). Chocolate and the brain: neurobiological impact of cocoa flavanols on cognition and behavior. *Neuroscience & Biobehavioral Reviews, 37*(10), 2445-2453.

Miller, K. B., Hurst, W. J., Payne, M. J., Stuart, D. A., Apgar, J., Sweigart, D. S., & Ou, B. (2008). Impact of alkalization on the antioxidant and flavanol content of commercial cocoa powders. *Journal of agricultural and food chemistry, 56*(18), 8527-8533.

Chapter 3. Wine, or Grapes?

"The French Paradox"

Renaud, S. D., & de Lorgeril, M. (1992). Wine, alcohol, platelets, and the French paradox for coronary heart disease. *The Lancet, 339*(8808), 1523-1526.

Ruf, J. C. (2003). Overview of epidemiological studies on wine, health and mortality. *Drugs under experimental and clinical research, 29*(5-6), 173-179.

Low to moderate consumption of wine benefits cognitive ability

Letenneur, L. (2004). Risk of dementia and alcohol and wine consumption: a review of recent results. *Biological research, 37*(2), 189-193.

Lemeshow, S., Letenneur, L., Dartigues, J. F., Lafont, S., Orgogozo, J. M., & Commenges, D. (1998). Illustration of analysis taking into account complex survey considerations: the association between wine consumption and dementia in the

PAQUID study. *American Journal of Epidemiology*, *148*(3), 298-306.

Ruitenberg, A., van Swieten, J. C., Witteman, J. C., Mehta, K. M., van Duijn, C. M., Hofman, A., & Breteler, M. M. (2002). Alcohol consumption and risk of dementia: the Rotterdam Study. *The Lancet*, *359*(9303), 281-286.

Johansen, D., Friis, K., Skovenborg, E., & Grønbæk, M. (2006). Food buying habits of people who buy wine or beer: cross sectional study. *Bmj*, *332*(7540), 519-522.

Paschall, M., & Lipton, R. I. (2005). Wine preference and related health determinants in a US national sample of young adults. *Drug and alcohol dependence*, *78*(3), 339-344.

Wang, J., Ho, L., Zhao, Z., Seror, I., Humala, N., Dickstein, D. L., ... & Pasinetti, G. M. (2006). Moderate consumption of Cabernet Sauvignon attenuates Aβ neuropathology in a mouse model of Alzheimer's disease. *The FASEB Journal*, *20*(13), 2313-2320.

Corona, G., Vauzour, D., Hercelin, J., Williams, C. M., & Spencer, J. P. (2013). Phenolic acid intake, delivered via moderate champagne wine consumption, improves spatial working memory via the modulation of hippocampal and cortical protein expression/activation. *Antioxidants & redox signaling*, *19*(14), 1676-1689.

Martínez-Huélamo, M., Rodríguez-Morató, J., Boronat, A., & de la Torre, R. (2017). Modulation of Nrf2 by Olive Oil and Wine Polyphenols and Neuroprotection. *Antioxidants*, *6*(4), 73.

Wine, rather than beer and spirits, is good

Ruf, J. C. (2003). Overview of epidemiological studies on wine, health and mortality. *Drugs under experimental and clinical research*, *29*(5-6), 173-179.

Lindsay, J., Laurin, D., Verreault, R., Hébert, R., Helliwell, B., Hill, G. B., & McDowell, I. (2002). Risk factors for Alzheimer's disease: a prospective analysis from the Canadian Study of Health and Aging. *American journal of epidemiology*, *156*(5), 445-453.

Heavy drinking, irrespective of what one drinks, is bad

Lu, Y. L., & Richardson, H. N. (2014). Alcohol, stress hormones, and the prefrontal cortex: a proposed pathway to the dark side of addiction. *Neuroscience*, *277*, 139-151.

Thayer, J. F., Hall, M., Sollers, J. J., & Fischer, J. E. (2006). Alcohol use, urinary cortisol, and heart rate variability in apparently healthy men: evidence for impaired inhibitory control of the HPA axis in heavy drinkers. *International Journal of Psychophysiology*, *59*(3), 244-250.

Wu, D., & Cederbaum, A. I. (2003). Alcohol, oxidative stress, and free radical damage. *Alcohol Research and Health*, *27*, 277-284.

Das, S. K., & Vasudevan, D. M. (2007). Alcohol-induced oxidative stress. *Life sciences*, *81*(3), 177-187.

Finn, P. R., Justus, A., Mazas, C., & Steinmetz, J. E. (1999). Working memory, executive processes and the effects of alcohol on Go/No-Go learning: testing a model of behavioral regulation and impulsivity. *Psychopharmacology*, *146*(4), 465-472.

González-Reimers, E., Santolaria-Fernández, F., Martín-González, M. C., Fernández-Rodríguez, C. M., & Quintero-Platt, G. (2014). Alcoholism: a systemic proinflammatory condition. *World Journal of Gastroenterology: WJG*, *20*(40), 14660.

Goodlett, C. R., & Horn, K. H. (2001). Mechanisms of alcohol-induced damage to the developing nervous system. *Alcohol research and health*, *25*(3), 175-184.

Lieber, C. S. (2003). Relationships between nutrition, alcohol use, and liver disease. *Alcohol Research and Health*, *27*, 220-231.

van den Berg, H., van der Gaag, M., & Hendriks, H. (2002). Influence of lifestyle on vitamin bioavailability. *International journal for vitamin and nutrition research*, *72*(1), 53-59.

Hauser, S. R., Getachew, B., Taylor, R. E., & Tizabi, Y. (2011). Alcohol induced depressive-like behavior is associated with a reduction in hippocampal BDNF. *Pharmacology Biochemistry and Behavior*, *100*(2), 253-258.

Briones, T. L., & Woods, J. (2013). Chronic binge-like alcohol consumption in adolescence causes depression-like symptoms possibly mediated by the effects of BDNF on neurogenesis. *Neuroscience, 254*, 324-334.

Resnicoff, M., Rubini, M., Baserga, R., & Rubin, R. (1994). Ethanol inhibits insulin-like growth factor-1-mediated signalling and proliferation of C6 rat glioblastoma cells. *Laboratory investigation; a journal of technical methods and pathology, 71*(5), 657-662.

Women are more susceptible to the harmful effects of alcohol

Di Castelnuovo, A., Costanzo, S., Bagnardi, V., Donati, M. B., Iacoviello, L., & De Gaetano, G. (2006). Alcohol dosing and total mortality in men and women: an updated meta-analysis of 34 prospective studies. *Archives of internal medicine, 166*(22), 2437-2445.

National Institute on Alcohol Abuse and Alcoholism. What Is A Standard Drink? Available at https://www.niaaa.nih.gov/ alcohol-health/overview-alcohol-consumption/what-standard-drink (last accessed 2018-01-12)

Gordon, T., & Doyle, J. T. (1987). Drinking and mortality: the Albany Study. *American Journal of Epidemiology, 125*(2), 263-270.

Red wines are better than white ones

German, J. B., & Walzem, R. L. (2000). The health benefits of wine. *Annual review of nutrition, 20*(1), 561-593.

Opie, L. H., & Lecour, S. (2007). The red wine hypothesis: from concepts to protective signalling molecules. *European heart journal, 28*(14), 1683-1693.

Zhao, B., & Hall, C.A. (2008). Composition and antioxidant activity of raisin extracts obtained from various solvents. *Food Chem.* 108, 511–518.

Red wine versus grapes, which to choose?

Durak, İ., Avci, A., Kagmaz, M., Buyukkoqak, S., Burak Simen, M. Y., Elgun, S., & Serdar Ozturk, H. (1999). Comparison of antioxidant potentials of red wine, white wine, grape juice and alcohol. *Current medical research and opinion, 15*(4), 316-320.

Vinson, J. A., Teufel, K., & Wu, N. (2001). Red wine, dealcoholized red wine, and especially grape juice, inhibit atherosclerosis in a hamster model. *Atherosclerosis, 156*(1), 67-72.

Chapter 4. The Benefit of 10 Cups of Green Tea

Green tea for cancer

Green tea story: adapated from Cancer Survivor Story. Available https://www.groundgreentea.com/content/colon-cancer-survivor-story-green-tea-benefits (last accessed 2017-12-04)

Fujiki, H., Suganuma, M., Imai, K., & Nakachi, K. (2002). Green tea: cancer preventive beverage and/or drug. *Cancer letters*, *188*(1), 9-13.

Goto, T., Yoshida, Y., Kiso, M., & Nagashima, H. (1996). Simultaneous analysis of individual catechins and caffeine in green tea. *Journal of Chromatography A*, *749*(1-2), 295-299.

Zaveri, N. T. (2006). Green tea and its polyphenolic catechins: medicinal uses in cancer and noncancer applications. *Life sciences*, *78*(18), 2073-2080.

Yang, C. S., Ju, J., Lu, G., Xiao, H., Hao, X., Sang, S., & Lambert, J. D. (2008). Cancer prevention by tea and tea polyphenols. *Asia Pacific journal of clinical nutrition*, *17*(Suppl 1), 245.

Serafini, M., Del Rio, D., Yao, D.N., et al. (2011). Health Benefits of Tea. In: Benzie IFF, Wachtel-Galor S, editors. *Herbal Medicine: Biomolecular and Clinical Aspects*. 2nd edition. Boca Raton (FL): CRC Press/Taylor & Francis. Chapter 12.

Oz, H. S. (2017). Chronic Inflammatory Diseases and Green Tea Polyphenols. *Nutrients*, *9*(6), 561.

Tea benefits cognitive functions

Yang, C. S., Ju, J., Lu, G., Xiao, H., Hao, X., Sang, S., & Lambert, J. D. (2008). Cancer prevention by tea and tea polyphenols. *Asia Pacific journal of clinical nutrition*, *17*(Suppl 1), 245.

Checkoway, H., Powers, K., Smith-Weller, T., Franklin, G. M., Longstreth Jr, W. T., & Swanson, P. D. (2002). Parkinson's disease risks associated with cigarette smoking, alcohol consumption, and caffeine intake. *American journal of epidemiology*, *155*(8), 732-738.

Nurk, E., Refsum, H., Drevon, C. A., Tell, G. S., Nygaard, H. A., Engedal, K., & Smith, A. D. (2009). Intake of flavonoid-rich wine, tea, and chocolate by elderly men and women is associated with better cognitive test performance. *The Journal of nutrition*, *139*(1), 120-127.

Why green tea is better than black and oolong tea

Yang, C. S., Ju, J., Lu, G., Xiao, H., Hao, X., Sang, S., & Lambert, J. D. (2008). Cancer prevention by tea and tea polyphenols. *Asia Pacific journal of clinical nutrition*, *17*(Suppl 1), 245.

Peterson, J., Dwyer, J., Bhagwat, S., Haytowitz, D., Holden, J., Eldridge, A. L., ... & Aladesanmi, J. (2005). Major flavonoids in dry tea. *Journal of Food Composition and Analysis*, *18*(6), 487-501.

Noguchi-Shinohara, M., Yuki, S., Dohmoto, C., Ikeda, Y., Samuraki, M., Iwasa, K., ... & Yamada, M. (2014). Consumption of green tea, but not black tea or coffee, is associated with reduced risk of cognitive decline. *PLoS One*, *9*(5), e96013.

Coffee is better restricted

Crippa, A., Discacciati, A., Larsson, S. C., Wolk, A., & Orsini, N. (2014). Coffee consumption and mortality from all causes, cardiovascular disease, and cancer: a dose-response meta-analysis. *American journal of epidemiology*, *180*(8), 763-775.

Kim, Y. S., Kwak, S. M., & Myung, S. K. (2015). Caffeine intake from coffee or tea and cognitive disorders: a meta-analysis of observational studies. *Neuroepidemiology*, *44*(1), 51-63.

US Department of Health and Human Services. (2015). *2015–2020 dietary guidelines for Americans*. Washington (DC): USDA.

Barone, J. J., & Roberts, H. R. (1996). Caffeine consumption. *Food and Chemical Toxicology*, *34*(1), 119-129.

Custodero, C., Valiani, V., Agosti, P., Schilardi, A., D'Introno, A., Lozupone, M., ... & Sabbà, C. (2017). Dietary patterns, foods, and food groups: relation to late-life cognitive disorders. *Official Journal of the Italian Society of Gerontology and Geriatrics*, 78.

al'Absi, M., & LOVALLO, W.R. (2004). Caffeine effects on the human stress axis. In A. Nehlig (Ed.), *Coffee, tea, chocolate and the brain*, (pp. 113-131). Boca Raton, FL:CRC. Press LLC.

Solfrizzi, V., Panza, F., Imbimbo, B. P., D'Introno, A., Galluzzo, L., Gandin, C., ... & Di Carlo, A. (2015). Coffee consumption habits and the risk of mild cognitive impairment: the Italian

Longitudinal Study on Aging. *Journal of Alzheimer's Disease*, *47*(4), 889-899.

Chapter 5. Berry Everyday

Berries enhance cognitive functions

Devore, E. E., Kang, J. H., Breteler, M., & Grodstein, F. (2012). Dietary intakes of berries and flavonoids in relation to cognitive decline. *Annals of neurology*, *72*(1), 135-143.

Krikorian, R., Shidler, M. D., Nash, T. A., Kalt, W., Vinqvist-Tymchuk, M. R., Shukitt-Hale, B., & Joseph, J. A. (2010). Blueberry supplementation improves memory in older adults. *Journal of agricultural and food chemistry*, *58*(7), 3996-4000.

Nilsson, A., Salo, I., Plaza, M., & Björck, I. (2017). Effects of a mixed berry beverage on cognitive functions and cardiometabolic risk markers; A randomized cross-over study in healthy older adults. *PloS one*, *12*(11), e0188173.

Berries are among the highest-ranked antioxidants

Ovaskainen, M. L., Törrönen, R., Koponen, J. M., Sinkko, H., Hellström, J., Reinivuo, H., & Mattila, P. (2008). Dietary intake and major food sources of polyphenols in Finnish adults. *The Journal of Nutrition*, *138*(3), 562-566.

Neto, C.C., Vinson, J.A. (2011). Cranberry. In: Benzie IFF, Wachtel-Galor S, editors. *Herbal Medicine: Biomolecular and Clinical Aspects*. 2nd edition. Boca Raton (FL): CRC Press/Taylor & Francis. Chapter 6.

Wu, X., Beecher, G. R., Holden, J. M., Haytowitz, D. B., Gebhardt, S. E., & Prior, R. L. (2004). Lipophilic and hydrophilic antioxidant capacities of common foods in the United States. *Journal of agricultural and food chemistry*, *52*(12), 4026-4037.

Forbes-Hernandez, T. Y., Gasparrini, M., Afrin, S., Bompadre, S., Mezzetti, B., Quiles, J. L., ... & Battino, M. (2016). The healthy effects of strawberry polyphenols: which strategy behind antioxidant capacity?. *Critical reviews in food science and nutrition*, *56*(sup1), S46-S59.

Tavares, L., Figueira, I., McDougall, G. J., Vieira, H. L., Stewart, D., Alves, P. M., ... & Santos, C. N. (2013). Neuroprotective effects of digested polyphenols from wild blackberry species. *European journal of nutrition*, *52*(1), 225-236.

Harrison, F. E., & May, J. M. (2009). Vitamin C function in the brain: vital role of the ascorbate transporter SVCT2. *Free Radical Biology and Medicine*, *46*(6), 719-730.

Travica, N., Ried, K., Sali, A., Scholey, A., Hudson, I., & Pipingas, A. (2017). Vitamin C Status and Cognitive Function: A Systematic Review. *Nutrients*, *9*(9), 960.

Péneau, S., Galan, P., Jeandel, C., Ferry, M., Andreeva, V., Hercberg, S., ... & SU. VI. MAX 2 Research Group. (2011). Fruit and vegetable intake and cognitive function in the SU. VI. MAX 2 prospective study. *The American journal of clinical nutrition*, *94*(5), 1295-1303.

Hemilä, H. (2017). Vitamin C and Infections. *Nutrients*, *9*(4), 339.

Harrison, F. E. (2012). A critical review of vitamin C for the prevention of age-related cognitive decline and Alzheimer's disease. *Journal of Alzheimer's Disease*, *29*(4), 711-726.

Rai, A. R., Madhyastha, S., Rao, G. M., Rai, R., & Sahu, S. S. (2013). A comparison of resveratrol and vitamin C therapy on expression of BDNF in stressed rat brain homogenate. *IOSR Journal of Pharmacy*, 10, 22-27.

Huang, H., Chen, G., Liao, D., Zhu, Y., & Xue, X. (2016). Effects of berries consumption on cardiovascular risk factors: a meta-analysis with trial sequential analysis of randomized controlled trials. *Scientific reports*, *6*, 23625.

Alvarez-Suarez, J. M., Giampieri, F., Tulipani, S., Casoli, T., Di Stefano, G., González-Paramás, A. M., ... & Bompadre, S. (2014). One-month strawberry-rich anthocyanin supplementation ameliorates cardiovascular risk, oxidative stress markers and platelet activation in humans. *The Journal of nutritional biochemistry*, *25*(3), 289-294.

Grapes and tomatoes are also berries

Martí, R., Roselló, S., & Cebolla-Cornejo, J. (2016). Tomato as a source of carotenoids and polyphenols targeted to cancer prevention. *Cancers*, *8*(6), 58.

Kaulmann, A., & Bohn, T. (2014). Carotenoids, inflammation, and oxidative stress—implications of cellular signaling pathways and relation to chronic disease prevention. *Nutrition research*, *34*(11), 907-929.

Agarwal, S., & Rao, A. V. (2000). Tomato lycopene and its role in human health and chronic diseases. *Canadian Medical Association Journal*, *163*(6), 739-744.

Story, E. N., Kopec, R. E., Schwartz, S. J., & Harris, G. K. (2010). An update on the health effects of tomato lycopene. *Annual review of food science and technology*, *1*, 189-210.

Burton-Freeman, B., & Reimers, K. (2011). Tomato consumption and health: emerging benefits. *American Journal of Lifestyle Medicine*, *5*(2), 182-191.

Iwasawa, H., Morita, E., Yui, S., & Yamazaki, M. (2011). Anti-oxidant effects of kiwi fruit in vitro and in vivo. *Biological and Pharmaceutical Bulletin*, *34*(1), 128-134.

Pinelli, P., Romani, A., Fierini, E., Remorini, D., & Agati, G. (2013). Characterisation of the Polyphenol Content in the Kiwifruit (Actinidia deliciosa) Exocarp for the Calibration of a Fruit-sorting Optical Sensor. *Phytochemical Analysis*, 24(5), 460-466.

Chapter 6. Olives, for Peace and (Cognitive) Power

Olives story. Kerényi, Karl (1951). *The Gods of the Greeks*. London, England: Thames and Hudson

Olives are rich in polyphenols and MUFA

https://www.ars.usda.gov/northeast-area/beltsville-md/
beltsville-human-nutrition-research-center/nutrient-data-
laboratory/

Tangney, C. C., & Rasmussen, H. E. (2013). Polyphenols, inflammation, and cardiovascular disease. *Current atherosclerosis reports*, 15(5), 324.

MUFA, a good fat

Gillingham, L. G., Harris-Janz, S., & Jones, P. J. (2011). Dietary monounsaturated fatty acids are protective against metabolic syndrome and cardiovascular disease risk factors. *Lipids*, *46*(3), 209-228.

Bonanome, A., Pagnan, A., Biffanti, S., Opportuno, A., Sorgato, F., Dorella, M., ... & Ursini, F. (1992). Effect of dietary monounsaturated and polyunsaturated fatty acids on the susceptibility of plasma low density lipoproteins to oxidative modification. *Arteriosclerosis, Thrombosis, and Vascular Biology*, *12*(4), 529-533.

Carrillo, C., Cavia, M. D. M., & Alonso-Torre, S. (2012). Role of oleic acid in immune system; mechanism of action; a review. *Nutricion hospitalaria*, *27*(4).

Dumas, J.A., Bunn, J.Y., Nickerson, J., Crain, K.I., Ebenstein, D.B., Tarleton, E.K., et al., 2016. Dietary saturated fat and monounsaturated fat have reversible effects on brain function and the secretion of pro-inflammatory cytokines in young women. *Metabolism* 65 (10), 1582–1588.

Solfrizzi, V., Colacicco, A. M., D'Introno, A., Capurso, C., Torres, F., Rizzo, C., ... & Panza, F. (2006). Dietary intake of unsaturated fatty acids and age-related cognitive decline: a 8.5-year follow-up of the Italian Longitudinal Study on Aging. *Neurobiology of aging*, *27*(11), 1694-1704.

Zamroziewicz, M. K., Talukdar, M. T., Zwilling, C. E., & Barbey, A. K. (2017). Nutritional status, brain network organization, and general intelligence. *NeuroImage*, *161*, 241-250.

Samieri, C., Grodstein, F., Rosner, B. A., Kang, J. H., Cook, N. R., Manson, J. E., ... & Okereke, O. I. (2013). Mediterranean diet and cognitive function in older age: results from the Women's Health Study. *Epidemiology (Cambridge, Mass.)*, *24*(4), 490.

Olive oil enhances cognitive functions

Berr, C., Portet, F., Carriere, I., Akbaraly, T. N., Feart, C., Gourlet, V., ... & Ritchie, K. (2009). Olive oil and cognition: results from the three-city study. *Dementia and geriatric cognitive disorders*, *28*(4), 357-364.

Valls-Pedret, C., Lamuela-Raventós, R. M., Medina-Remón, A., Quintana, M., Corella, D., Pintó, X., ... & Ros, E. (2012). Polyphenol-rich foods in the Mediterranean diet are associated with better cognitive function in elderly subjects at high cardiovascular risk. *Journal of Alzheimer's disease*, *29*(4), 773-782.

Martinez-Lapiscina, E. H., Clavero, P., Toledo, E., San Julian, B., Sanchez-Tainta, A., Corella, D., ... & Martinez-Gonzalez, M. A. (2013). Virgin olive oil supplementation and long-term cognition: the PREDIMED-NAVARRA randomized, trial. *The journal of nutrition, health & aging*, *17*(6), 544-552.

Extra virgin olive oil is preferred

Cicerale, S., Lucas, L. J., & Keast, R. S. J. (2012). Antimicrobial, antioxidant and anti-inflammatory phenolic activities in extra virgin olive oil. *Current opinion in biotechnology*, *23*(2), 129-135.

Casas R, Estruch R, Sacanella E. (2017) The protective effects of extra virgin olive oil on immune-mediated inflammatory responses. *Endocr Metab Immune Disord Drug Targets*. 2017 Nov 13. doi: 10.2174/1871530317666171114115632.

Valls-Pedret, C., Sala-Vila, A., Serra-Mir, M., Corella, D., de la Torre, R., Martínez-González, M. Á., ... & Estruch, R. (2015). Mediterranean diet and age-related cognitive decline: a randomized clinical trial. *JAMA internal medicine*, *175*(7), 1094-1103.

Chapter 7. Nuts: Only Skin-deep?

Nuts enhance cognitive functions

Arab, L., & Ang, A. (2015). A cross sectional study of the association between walnut consumption and cognitive function among adult us populations represented in NHANES. *The journal of nutrition, health & aging, 19*(3), 284.

O'BRIEN, J., Okereke, O., Devore, E., Rosner, B., Breteler, M., & Grodstein, F. (2014). Long-term intake of nuts in relation to cognitive function in older women. *The journal of nutrition, health & aging, 18*(5), 496.

Nuts are among the highest-ranked antioxidants

Hernández-Alonso, P., Camacho-Barcia, L., Bulló, M., & Salas-Salvadó, J. (2017). Nuts and Dried Fruits: An Update of Their Beneficial Effects on Type 2 Diabetes. *Nutrients, 9*(7), 673.

Vinson, J. A., & Cai, Y. (2012). Nuts, especially walnuts, have both antioxidant quantity and efficacy and exhibit significant potential health benefits. *Food & function, 3*(2), 134-140.

Wu, X., Beecher, G. R., Holden, J. M., Haytowitz, D. B., Gebhardt, S. E., & Prior, R. L. (2004). Lipophilic and hydrophilic antioxidant capacities of common foods in the United States. *Journal of agricultural and food chemistry, 52*(12), 4026-4037.

Why nuts are only skin-deep

Milbury, P. E., Chen, C. Y., Dolnikowski, G. G., & Blumberg, J. B. (2006). Determination of flavonoids and phenolics and their distribution in almonds. *Journal of Agricultural and Food Chemistry*, *54*(14), 5027-5033.

Chen, C. Y., Milbury, P. E., Lapsley, K., & Blumberg, J. B. (2005). Flavonoids from almond skins are bioavailable and act synergistically with vitamins C and E to enhance hamster and human LDL resistance to oxidation. *The journal of nutrition*, *135*(6), 1366-1373.

Lou, H., Yuan, H., Ma, B., Ren, D., Ji, M., & Oka, S. (2004). Polyphenols from peanut skins and their free radical-scavenging effects. *Phytochemistry*, *65*(16), 2391-2399.

Nuts are calories dense, yet do not cause weight gain

Boulangé, C. L., Neves, A. L., Chilloux, J., Nicholson, J. K., & Dumas, M. E. (2016). Impact of the gut microbiota on inflammation, obesity, and metabolic disease. *Genome medicine*, *8*(1), 42.

Flint, H. J. (2012). The impact of nutrition on the human microbiome. *Nutrition reviews*, *70*(s1).

Flint, H. J., Scott, K. P., Duncan, S. H., Louis, P., & Forano, E. (2012). Microbial degradation of complex carbohydrates in the gut. *Gut microbes*, *3*(4), 289-306.

Maukonen, J., & Saarela, M. (2015). Human gut microbiota: does diet matter?. *Proceedings of the Nutrition Society*, *74*(1), 23-36.

Schroeder, F. A., Lin, C. L., Crusio, W. E., & Akbarian, S. (2007). Antidepressant-like effects of the histone deacetylase inhibitor, sodium butyrate, in the mouse. *Biological psychiatry*, *62*(1), 55-64.

Kaczmarczyk, M. M., Miller, M. J., & Freund, G. G. (2012). The health benefits of dietary fiber: beyond the usual suspects of type 2 diabetes mellitus, cardiovascular disease and colon cancer. *Metabolism*, *61*(8), 1058-1066.

Khan, N. A., Raine, L. B., Drollette, E. S., Scudder, M. R., Kramer, A. F., & Hillman, C. H. (2014). Dietary Fiber Is Positively Associated with Cognitive Control among Prepubertal Children, 2. *The Journal of nutrition*, *145*(1), 143-149.

Daily 30–60 g of nuts are recommended

Vinson, J. A., & Cai, Y. (2012). Nuts, especially walnuts, have both antioxidant quantity and efficacy and exhibit significant potential health benefits. *Food & function*, *3*(2), 134-140.

Ros, E. (2010). Health benefits of nut consumption. *Nutrients*, *2*(7), 652-682.

Bes-Rastrollo M, Sabaté J, Gómez-Gracia E, Alonso A, Martínez JA, Martínez-González MA. (2007). Nut consumption and weight gain in a Mediterranean cohort: The SUN study. *Obesity (Silver Spring)*. 15(1):107-16.

Willis, L. M., Shukitt-Hale, B., Cheng, V., & Joseph, J. A. (2008). Dose-dependent effects of walnuts on motor and cognitive function in aged rats. *British journal of nutrition*, *101*(8), 1140-1144.

Pribis, P., Bailey, R. N., Russell, A. A., Kilsby, M. A., Hernandez, M., Craig, W. J., ... & Sabatè, J. (2012). Effects of walnut consumption on cognitive performance in young adults. *British journal of nutrition*, *107*(9), 1393-1401.

Pribis, P., & Shukitt-Hale, B. (2014). Cognition: the new frontier for nuts and berries. *The American journal of clinical nutrition*, *100*(Supplement 1), 347S-352S.

PUFA and its two families: omega-3 versus omega-6

Delarue, J. O. C. P., Matzinger, O., Binnert, C., Schneiter, P., Chiolero, R., & Tappy, L. (2003). Fish oil prevents the adrenal activation elicited by mental stress in healthy men. *Diabetes & metabolism*, *29*(3), 289-295.

Michaeli, B., Berger, M. M., Revelly, J. P., Tappy, L., & Chioléro, R. (2007). Effects of fish oil on the neuro-endocrine responses to an endotoxin challenge in healthy volunteers. *Clinical nutrition*, *26*(1), 70-77.

Larrieu, T., Hilal, L. M., Fourrier, C., De Smedt-Peyrusse, V., Sans, N., Capuron, L., & Laye, S. (2014). Nutritional omega-3 modulates neuronal morphology in the prefrontal cortex along with depression-related behaviour through corticosterone secretion. *Translational psychiatry*, *4*(9), e437.

Mocking, R. J., Ruhé, H. G., Assies, J., Lok, A., Koeter, M. W., Visser, I., ... & Schene, A. H. (2013). Relationship between the hypothalamic–pituitary–adrenal-axis and fatty acid metabolism in recurrent depression. *Psychoneuroendocrinology*, *38*(9), 1607-1617.

Chen, H. F., & Su, H. M. (2013). Exposure to a maternal n-3 fatty acid-deficient diet during brain development provokes excessive hypothalamic–pituitary–adrenal axis responses to stress and behavioral indices of depression and anxiety in male rat offspring later in life. *The Journal of nutritional biochemistry*, *24*(1), 70-80.

Kiecolt-Glaser, J. K., Belury, M. A., Andridge, R., Malarkey, W. B., & Glaser, R. (2011). Omega-3 supplementation lowers inflammation and anxiety in medical students: a randomized controlled trial. *Brain, behavior, and immunity*, *25*(8), 1725-1734.

Li, K., Huang, T., Zheng, J., Wu, K., & Li, D. (2014). Effect of marine-derived n-3 polyunsaturated fatty acids on C-reactive protein, interleukin 6 and tumor necrosis factor α: a meta-analysis. *PloS one*, *9*(2), e88103.

Simopoulos, A. P. (2002). Omega-3 fatty acids in inflammation and autoimmune diseases. *Journal of the American College of Nutrition*, *21*(6), 495-505.

Ouchi, N., & Walsh, K. (2007). Adiponectin as an anti-inflammatory factor. *Clinica chimica acta*, *380*(1), 24-30.

Kuszewski JC, Wong RHX, Howe PRC. (2017) Effects of Long-Chain Omega-3 Polyunsaturated Fatty Acids on Endothelial Vasodilator Function and Cognition-Are They Interrelated? *Nutrients*. 2017 May 12;9(5). pii: E487. doi: 10.3390/nu9050487.

Zanetti, M., Grillo, A., Losurdo, P., Panizon, E., Mearelli, F., Cattin, L., ... & Carretta, R. (2015). Omega-3 polyunsaturated fatty acids: structural and functional effects on the vascular wall. *BioMed research international*, *2015*.

Weiser, M. J., Butt, C. M., & Mohajeri, M. H. (2016). Docosahexaenoic acid and cognition throughout the lifespan. *Nutrients*, *8*(2), 99.

Yurko-Mauro, K., Alexander, D. D., & Van Elswyk, M. E. (2015). Docosahexaenoic acid and adult memory: a systematic review and meta-analysis. *PLoS One*, *10*(3), e0120391.

Bazinet, R. P., & Layé, S. (2014). Polyunsaturated fatty acids and their metabolites in brain function and disease. *Nature Reviews Neuroscience*, *15*(12), 771-785.

Flock, M. R., Harris, W. S., & Kris-Etherton, P. M. (2013). Long-chain omega-3 fatty acids: time to establish a dietary reference intake. *Nutrition reviews*, *71*(10), 692-707.

Beltz, B. S., Tlusty, M. F., Benton, J. L., & Sandeman, D. C. (2007). Omega-3 fatty acids upregulate adult neurogenesis. *Neuroscience letters*, *415*(2), 154-158.

Takeuchi, T., Fukumoto, Y., & Harada, E. (2002). Influence of a dietary n-3 fatty acid deficiency on the cerebral catecholamine contents, EEG and learning ability in rat. *Behavioural brain research*, *131*(1), 193-203.

Minami, M., Kimura, S., Endo, T., Hamaue, N., Hirafuji, M., Togashi, H., ... & Kobayashi, T. (1997). Dietary docosahexaenoic acid increases cerebral acetylcholine levels and improves passive avoidance performance in stroke-prone spontaneously hypertensive rats. *Pharmacology biochemistry and behavior*, *58*(4), 1123-1129.

Hadjighassem, M., Kamalidehghan, B., Shekarriz, N., Baseerat, A., Molavi, N., Mehrpour, M., ... & Meng, G. Y. (2015). Oral consumption of α-linolenic acid increases serum BDNF levels in healthy adult humans. *Nutrition journal*, *14*(1), 20.

Wu, A., Ying, Z., & Gomez-Pinilla, F. (2008). Docosahexaenoic acid dietary supplementation enhances the effects of exercise on synaptic plasticity and cognition. *Neuroscience*, *155*(3), 751-759.

Rao, J. S., Ertley, R. N., Lee, H. J., DeMar Jr, J. C., Arnold, J. T., Rapoport, S. I., & Bazinet, R. P. (2007). n-3 polyunsaturated fatty acid deprivation in rats decreases frontal cortex BDNF via a p38 MAPK-dependent mechanism. *Molecular psychiatry*, *12*(1), 36.

A target ratio of 1–2:1 of omega-6: omega-3 is preferred

Simopoulos, A. P. (2010). The omega-6/omega-3 fatty acid ratio: health implications. *Oléagineux, Corps gras, Lipides*, *17*(5), 267-275.

Simopoulos, A. P. (2011). Evolutionary Aspects of Diet: The Omega-6/Omega-3 Ratio and the Brain. *Molecular Neurobiology*.

Patterson, E., Wall, R., Fitzgerald, G. F., Ross, R. P., & Stanton, C. (2012). Health implications of high dietary omega-6 polyunsaturated fatty acids. *Journal of nutrition and metabolism*, *2012*.

Loef, M., & Walach, H. (2013). The omega-6/omega-3 ratio and dementia or cognitive decline: a systematic review on human studies and biological evidence. *Journal of nutrition in gerontology and geriatrics*, *32*(1), 1-23.

Blomhoff, R., Carlsen, M. H., Andersen, L. F., & Jacobs, D. R. (2006). Health benefits of nuts: potential role of antioxidants. *British Journal of Nutrition*, *96*(S2), S52-S60.

Jenkins, D. J. (2008). Fish oil and omega-3 fatty acids. *Canadian Medical Association. Journal*, *178*(2), 150.

Chapter 8. In Search of Coldwater, Fatty Fish

Valentine, R. C., & Valentine, D. L. (2009). *Omega-3 fatty acids and the DHA principle*. CRC press.

the best seafood in the world: Hokkaido Seafood Guide – Japan. Available at http://supersillytraveller.com/hokkaido-seafood-guide-japan/ (last visited 2017-12-12)

Seafood enhances cognitive performance

Arab, L. (2003). Biomarkers of fat and fatty acid intake. *The Journal of nutrition*, 133(3), 925S-932S.

Tan, Z. S., Harris, W. S., Beiser, A. S., Au, R., Himali, J. J., Debette, S., ... & Robins, S. J. (2012). Red blood cell omega-3 fatty acid levels and markers of accelerated brain aging. *Neurology*, *78*(9), 658-664.

Sørensen, L. B., Damsgaard, C. T., Dalskov, S. M., Petersen, R. A., Egelund, N., Dyssegaard, C. B., ... & Michaelsen, K. F. (2015). Diet-induced changes in iron and n-3 fatty acid status and associations with cognitive performance in 8–11-year-old Danish children: secondary analyses of the Optimal Well-Being, Development and Health for Danish Children through a Healthy New Nordic Diet School Meal Study. *British Journal of Nutrition*, *114*(10), 1623-1637.

Åberg, M. A., Åberg, N., Brisman, J., Sundberg, R., Winkvist, A., & Torén, K. (2009). Fish intake of Swedish male adolescents is a predictor of cognitive performance. *Acta paediatrica*, *98*(3), 555-560.

Morris, M. C., Evans, D. A., Tangney, C. C., Bienias, J. L., & Wilson, R. S. (2005). Fish consumption and cognitive decline with age in a large community study. *Archives of neurology*, *62*(12), 1849-1853.

Qin, B., Plassman, B. L., Edwards, L. J., Popkin, B. M., Adair, L. S., & Mendez, M. A. (2014). Fish intake is associated with slower cognitive decline in Chinese older adults. *The Journal of nutrition, 144*(10), 1579-1585.

Eating fish at least twice per week

Nurk, E., Drevon, C. A., Refsum, H., Solvoll, K., Vollset, S. E., Nygård, O., ... & Smith, A. D. (2007). Cognitive performance among the elderly and dietary fish intake: the Hordaland Health Study. *The American journal of clinical nutrition, 86*(5), 1470-1478.

US Department of Health and Human Services. (2015). *2015–2020 dietary guidelines for Americans*. Washington (DC): USDA.

The problem with fish

World Health Organization. (2007). Exposure to mercury: A major public health concern. *WHO, Public Health and Environment.*

EPA website, *Fish Consumption Advisories, General Information*. Available at: http://water.epa.gov/scitech/swguidance/fishshellfish/fishadvisories/general.cfm
(last accessed 2017/8/10)

Candela, M., Astiasaran, I., & Bello, J. (1998). Deep-fat frying modifies high-fat fish lipid fraction. *Journal of Agricultural and Food Chemistry*, *46*(7), 2793-2796.

A list of coldwater, fatty fish with low mercury contaminations

First appeared in Chen, C. (2017). *The Seed of Intelligence: Boost Your Baby's Developing Brain through Optimal Nutrition and Healthy Lifestyle*. London: Brain & Life Publishing

The problem with sushi and sashimi

Candela, M., Astiasaran, I., & Bello, J. (1998). Deep-fat frying modifies high-fat fish lipid fraction. *Journal of Agricultural and Food Chemistry*, *46*(7), 2793-2796.

EPA website, *Fish Consumption Advisories, General Information*. Available at: http://water.epa.gov/scitech/ swguidance/fishshellfish/fishadvisories/general.cfm (last accessed 2017/8/10)

Chapter 9. The Healthy Way (1): From "5 A Day" to "10 A Day"

Any food can be YOUR brain food

Lomagno, K. A., Hu, F., Riddell, L. J., Booth, A. O., Szymlek-Gay, E. A., Nowson, C. A., & Byrne, L. K. (2014). Increasing iron and zinc in pre-menopausal women and its effects on mood and cognition: a systematic review. *Nutrients*, *6*(11), 5117-5141.

For the introduction of iron, see *The Seed of Intelligence*

Patterns are that all matter: the healthy way

Kant, A. K. (1996). Indexes of overall diet quality: a review. *Journal of the American Dietetic Association*, *96*(8), 785-791.

Hu, F. B. (2002). Dietary pattern analysis: a new direction in nutritional epidemiology. *Current opinion in lipidology*, *13*(1), 3-9.

Alles, B., Samieri, C., Feart, C., Jutand, M. A., Laurin, D., & Barberger-Gateau, P. (2012). Dietary patterns: a novel approach to examine the link between nutrition and cognitive function in older individuals. *Nutrition research reviews*, *25*(2), 207-222.

Custodero, C., Valiani, V., Agosti, P., Schilardi, A., D'Introno, A., Lozupone, M., ... & Sabbà, C. (2017). Dietary patterns, foods, and food groups: relation to late-life cognitive disorders. *Official Journal of the Italian Society of Gerontology and Geriatrics*, 78.

Burrows, T., Goldman, S., Pursey, K., & Lim, R. (2017). Is there an association between dietary intake and academic achievement: a systematic review. *Journal of Human Nutrition and Dietetics*, *30*(2), 117-140.

Cohen, J. F., Gorski, M. T., Gruber, S. A., Kurdziel, L. B. F., & Rimm, E. B. (2016). The effect of healthy dietary consumption on executive cognitive functioning in children and adolescents: a systematic review. *British Journal of Nutrition*, *116*(6), 989-1000.

Correa-Burrows, P., Rodríguez, Y., Blanco, E., Gahagan, S., & Burrows, R. (2017). Snacking Quality Is Associated with Secondary School Academic Achievement and the Intention to Enroll in Higher Education: A Cross-Sectional Study in Adolescents from Santiago, Chile. *Nutrients*, *9*(5), 433.

Goetzel, R. Z., & Ozminkowski, R. J. (2008). The health and cost benefits of work site health-promotion programs. *Annu. Rev. Public Health*, *29*, 303-323.

van de Rest, O., Berendsen, A. A., Haveman-Nies, A., & de Groot, L. C. (2015). Dietary patterns, cognitive decline, and dementia: a systematic review. *Advances in nutrition: an international review journal*, *6*(2), 154-168.

Aridi, Y. S., Walker, J. L., & Wright, O. R. (2017). The association between the Mediterranean dietary pattern and cognitive health: a systematic review. *Nutrients*, *9*(7), 674.

Lichtenstein, A. H., Appel, L. J., Brands, M., Carnethon, M., Daniels, S., Franch, H. A., ... & Karanja, N. (2006). Diet and lifestyle recommendations revision 2006. *Circulation*, *114*(1), 82-96.

Martínez-González, M. A., & Sánchez-Villegas, A. (2016). Food patterns and the prevention of depression. *Proceedings of the Nutrition Society*, *75*(2), 139-146.

Katz, D. L., & Meller, S. (2014). Can we say what diet is best for health?. *Annual review of public health*, *35*, 83-103.

Vegetables and fruits: "5 A Day"

World Health Organization. (1990). Diet, nutrition and the prevention of chronic diseases: report of a WHO study group [meeting held in Geneva from 6-13 March 1989].

US Department of Health and Human Services. (2015). *2015–2020 dietary guidelines for Americans*. Washington (DC): USDA.

Portion size: NHS Choices. Rough guide - Fruit & vegetable portion sizes. Available https://www.nhs.uk/Livewell/5ADAY/Documents/Downloads/5ADAY_portion_guide.pdf
(last accessed 2018-01-05)

Pastor-Valero, M., Furlan-Viebig, R., Menezes, P. R., da Silva, S. A., Vallada, H., & Scazufca, M. (2014). Education and WHO recommendations for fruit and vegetable intake are associated with better cognitive function in a disadvantaged Brazilian elderly population: a population-based cross-sectional study. *PloS one*, *9*(4), e94042.

Wang, X., Ouyang, Y., Liu, J., Zhu, M., Zhao, G., Bao, W., & Hu, F. B. (2014). Fruit and vegetable consumption and mortality from all causes, cardiovascular disease, and cancer: systematic review and dose-response meta-analysis of prospective cohort studies. *Bmj*, *349*, g4490.

Riggs, N. R., Spruijt-Metz, D., Chou, C. P., & Pentz, M. A. (2012). Relationships between executive cognitive function and lifetime substance use and obesity-related behaviors in fourth grade youth. *Child Neuropsychology*, *18*(1), 1-11.

Hughes, T. F., Andel, R., Small, B. J., Borenstein, A. R., Mortimer, J. A., Wolk, A., ... & Gatz, M. (2010). Midlife fruit and vegetable consumption and risk of dementia in later life in Swedish twins. *The American journal of geriatric psychiatry*, *18*(5), 413-420.

From "5 A Day" to "10 A Day"

Aune, D., Giovannucci, E., Boffetta, P., Fadnes, L. T., Keum, N., Norat, T., ... & Tonstad, S. (2017). Fruit and vegetable intake and the risk of cardiovascular disease, total cancer and all-cause mortality–a systematic review and dose-response meta-analysis of prospective studies. *International Journal of Epidemiology*, 46(3):1029-1056.

Li, R., Scrdula, M., Bland, S., Mokdad, A., Bowman, B., & Nelson, D. (2000). Trends in fruit and vegetable consumption among adults in 16 US states: Behavioral Risk Factor Surveillance System, 1990-1996. *American Journal of Public Health*, *90*(5), 777.

Frank, B., & Gupta, S. (2005). A review of antioxidants and Alzheimer's disease. *Annals of Clinical Psychiatry*, *17*(4), 269-286.

Chapter 10. The Healthy Way (2): The Mediterranean Diet

Keys, A., Aravanis, C., Buchem, F. S. P., & Blackburn, H. (1981). The diet and all-causes death rate in the Seven Countries Study. *Lancet*, (8237), 58-61.

The Mediterranean diet dissected

Sofi, F., Macchi, C., Abbate, R., Gensini, G. F., & Casini, A. (2014). Mediterranean diet and health status: an updated meta-analysis and a proposal for a literature-based adherence score. *Public health nutrition*, *17*(12), 2769-2782.

Oldways Preservation and Exchange Trust. (2009). *The Mediterranean Diet Pyramid*. Available at https://oldwayspt.org/traditional-diets/mediterranean-diet (last accessed 2018-01-15)

Whole grains are healthier than refined ones

Ludwig, D. S. (2007). Clinical update: the low-glycaemic-index diet. *The Lancet*, *369*(9565), 890-892.

Steffen, L. M., Jacobs, D. R., Stevens, J., Shahar, E., Carithers, T., & Folsom, A. R. (2003). Associations of whole-grain, refined-grain, and fruit and vegetable consumption with risks of all-cause mortality and incident coronary artery disease and ischemic stroke: the Atherosclerosis Risk in Communities (ARIC) Study. *The American journal of clinical nutrition*, *78*(3), 383-390.

Aune, D., Norat, T., Romundstad, P., & Vatten, L. J. (2013). Whole grain and refined grain consumption and the risk of type 2 diabetes: a systematic review and dose–response meta-analysis of cohort studies. *European journal of epidemiology*, *28*(11), 845-858.

Campbell, G. J., Senior, A. M., & Bell-Anderson, K. S. (2017). Metabolic Effects of High Glycaemic Index Diets: A Systematic Review and Meta-Analysis of Feeding Studies in Mice and Rats. *Nutrients*, *9*(7), 646.

Seal, C. J., & Brownlee, I. A. (2015). Whole-grain foods and chronic disease: evidence from epidemiological and intervention studies. *Proceedings of the Nutrition Society*, *74*(3), 313-319.

One of the healthiest diets

Valls-Pedret, C., Lamuela-Raventós, R. M., Medina-Remón, A., Quintana, M., Corella, D., Pintó, X., ... & Ros, E. (2012). Polyphenol-rich foods in the Mediterranean diet are associated with better cognitive function in elderly subjects at high cardiovascular risk. *Journal of Alzheimer's disease*, *29*(4), 773-782.

Esposito, K., Nappo, F., Giugliano, F., Di Palo, C., Ciotola, M., Barbieri, M., ... & Giugliano, D. (2003). Meal modulation of circulating interleukin 18 and adiponectin concentrations in healthy subjects and in patients with type 2 diabetes mellitus. *The American journal of clinical nutrition*, *78*(6), 1135-1140.

Schwingshackl, L., & Hoffmann, G. (2015). Adherence to Mediterranean diet and risk of cancer: an updated systematic review and meta-analysis of observational studies. *Cancer medicine*, *4*(12), 1933-1947.

Schwingshackl, L., Missbach, B., König, J., & Hoffmann, G. (2015). Adherence to a Mediterranean diet and risk of diabetes: a systematic review and meta-analysis. *Public health nutrition*, *18*(7), 1292-1299.

Aridi, Y. S., Walker, J. L., & Wright, O. R. (2017). The association between the Mediterranean dietary pattern and cognitive health: a systematic review. *Nutrients*, *9*(7), 674.

Psaltopoulou, T., Sergentanis, T. N., Panagiotakos, D. B., Sergentanis, I. N., Kosti, R., & Scarmeas, N. (2013). Mediterranean diet, stroke, cognitive impairment, and depression: a meta-analysis. *Annals of neurology*, *74*(4), 580-591.

Pelletier, A., Barul, C., Féart, C., Helmer, C., Bernard, C., Periot, O., ... & Catheline, G. (2015). Mediterranean diet and preserved brain structural connectivity in older subjects. *Alzheimer's & Dementia*, *11*(9), 1023-1031.

Gu, Y., Brickman, A. M., Stern, Y., Habeck, C. G., Razlighi, Q. R., Luchsinger, J. A., ... & Scarmeas, N. (2015). Mediterranean diet and brain structure in a multiethnic elderly cohort. *Neurology*, *85*(20), 1744-1751.

Research within the Mediterranean area

Aridi, Y. S., Walker, J. L., & Wright, O. R. (2017). The association between the Mediterranean dietary pattern and cognitive health: a systematic review. *Nutrients*, *9*(7), 674.

Trichopoulou, A., Kyrozis, A., Rossi, M., Katsoulis, M., Trichopoulos, D., La Vecchia, C., & Lagiou, P. (2015). Mediterranean diet and cognitive decline over time in an elderly Mediterranean population. *European journal of nutrition*, *54*(8), 1311-1321.

Research outside the Mediterranean area

Tangney, C. C., Kwasny, M. J., Li, H., Wilson, R. S., Evans, D. A., & Morris, M. C. (2011). Adherence to a Mediterranean-type dietary pattern and cognitive decline in a community population. *The American journal of clinical nutrition*, *93*(3), 601-607.

Tsivgoulis, G., Judd, S., Letter, A. J., Alexandrov, A. V., Howard, G., Nahab, F., ... & Wadley, V. G. (2013). Adherence to a Mediterranean diet and risk of incident cognitive impairment. *Neurology*, *80*(18), 1684-1692.

Qin, B., Adair, L. S., Plassman, B. L., Batis, C., Edwards, L. J., Popkin, B. M., & Mendez, M. A. (2015). Dietary patterns and cognitive decline among Chinese older adults. *Epidemiology*, *26*(5), 758-768.

Morris, M. C., Tangney, C. C., Wang, Y., Sacks, F. M., Barnes, L. L., Bennett, D. A., & Aggarwal, N. T. (2015). MIND diet slows cognitive decline with aging. *Alzheimer's & dementia, 11*(9), 1015-1022.

"The way not taken" is not necessarily bad

US Department of Health and Human Services. (2015). 2015–2020 dietary guidelines for Americans. *Washington (DC): USDA.*

Micha, R., Wallace, S. K., & Mozaffarian, D. (2010). Red and processed meat consumption and risk of incident coronary heart disease, stroke, and diabetes mellitus. *Circulation, 121*(21), 2271-2283.

Staubo, S. C., Aakre, J. A., Vemuri, P., Syrjanen, J. A., Mielke, M. M., Geda, Y. E., ... & Jack, C. R. (2017). Mediterranean diet, micronutrients and macronutrients, and MRI measures of cortical thickness. *Alzheimer's & Dementia, 13*(2), 168-177.

Griffin, B. A. (2016). Eggs: good or bad?. *Proceedings of the Nutrition Society, 75*(3), 259-264.

Fernandez, M. L. (2016). Eggs and Health Special Issue. *Nutrients, 8,* 784

Zhao, X., Yuan, L., Feng, L., Xi, Y., Yu, H., Ma, W., ... & Xiao, R. (2015). Association of dietary intake and lifestyle pattern with mild cognitive impairment in the elderly. *The journal of nutrition, health & aging, 19*(2), 164.

Chapter 11. The Unhealthy Way: 4 Driving Forces

Four groups of brain junk food

US Department of Health and Human Services. (2015). 2015–2020 dietary guidelines for Americans. *Washington (DC): USDA.*

Custodero, C., Valiani, V., Agosti, P., Schilardi, A., D'Introno, A., Lozupone, M., ... & Sabbà, C. (2017). Dietary patterns, foods, and food groups: relation to late-life cognitive disorders. *Official Journal of the Italian Society of Gerontology and Geriatrics*, 78.

Jacka, F. N. (2017). Nutritional Psychiatry: Where to Next?. *EBioMedicine.* 17, 24–29.

Micha, R., Wallace, S. K., & Mozaffarian, D. (2010). Red and processed meat consumption and risk of incident coronary heart disease, stroke, and diabetes mellitus. *Circulation, 121*(21), 2271-2283.

Schulze, M. B., Manson, J. E., Willett, W. C., & Hu, F. B. (2003). Processed meat intake and incidence of type 2 diabetes in younger and middle-aged women. *Diabetologia, 46*(11), 1465-1473.

Guallar-Castillón, P., Rodríguez-Artalejo, F., Fornés, N. S., Banegas, J. R., Etxezarreta, P. A., Ardanaz, E., ... & Losada, A. (2007). Intake of fried foods is associated with obesity in the cohort of Spanish adults from the European Prospective

Investigation into Cancer and Nutrition. *The American journal of clinical nutrition*, *86*(1), 198-205.

Mozaffarian, D., Hao, T., Rimm, E. B., Willett, W. C., & Hu, F. B. (2011). Changes in diet and lifestyle and long-term weight gain in women and men. *New England Journal of Medicine*, *364*(25), 2392-2404.

Odegaard, A. O., Koh, W. P., Yuan, J. M., Gross, M. D., & Pereira, M. A. (2012). Western-style fast food intake and cardio-metabolic risk in an eastern country. *Circulation*, CIRCULATIONAHA-111.

Lopez-Garcia, E., Schulze, M. B., Fung, T. T., Meigs, J. B., Rifai, N., Manson, J. E., & Hu, F. B. (2004). Major dietary patterns are related to plasma concentrations of markers of inflammation and endothelial dysfunction. *The American journal of clinical nutrition*, *80*(4), 1029-1035.

Bayer-Carter, J. L., Green, P. S., Montine, T. J., VanFossen, B., Baker, L. D., Watson, G. S., ... & Tsai, E. (2011). Diet intervention and cerebrospinal fluid biomarkers in amnestic mild cognitive impairment. *Archives of neurology*, *68*(6), 743-752.

Smithers, L. G., Golley, R. K., Mittinty, M. N., Brazionis, L., Northstone, K., Emmett, P., & Lynch, J. W. (2012). Dietary patterns at 6, 15 and 24 months of age are associated with IQ at 8 years of age. *European journal of epidemiology*, *27*(7), 525-535.

Smithers, L. G., Golley, R. K., Mittinty, M. N., Brazionis, L., Northstone, K., Emmett, P., & Lynch, J. W. (2013). Do dietary trajectories between infancy and toddlerhood influence IQ in childhood and adolescence? Results from a prospective birth cohort study. *PloS one*, *8*(3), e58904.

Feinstein, L., Sabates, R., Sorhaindo, A., Rogers, I., Herrick, D., Northstone, K., & Emmett, P. (2008). Dietary patterns related to attainment in school: the importance of early eating patterns. *Journal of Epidemiology & Community Health*, *62*(8), 734-739.

Nyaradi, A., Li, J., Hickling, S., Whitehouse, A. J., Foster, J. K., & Oddy, W. H. (2013). Diet in the early years of life influences cognitive outcomes at 10 years: a prospective cohort study. *Acta Paediatrica*, *102*(12), 1165-1173.

Ames, S. L., Kisbu-Sakarya, Y., Reynolds, K. D., Boyle, S., Cappelli, C., Cox, M. G., ... & Stacy, A. W. (2014). Inhibitory control effects in adolescent binge eating and consumption of sugar-sweetened beverages and snacks. *Appetite*, *81*, 180-192.

The unhealthy way dissected

Monteiro, C. A., Levy, R. B., Claro, R. M., de Castro, I. R. R., & Cannon, G. (2010). Increasing consumption of ultra-processed foods and likely impact on human health: evidence from Brazil. *Public health nutrition*, *14*(1), 5-13.

Choe, E., & Min, D. B. (2007). Chemistry of deep-fat frying oils. *Journal of food science*, *72*(5).

Driving force No.1: saturated fat

Kalmijn, S., Launer, L. J., Ott, A., Witteman, J., Hofman, A., & Breteler, M. (1997). Dietary fat intake and the risk of incident dementia in the Rotterdam Study. *Annals of neurology*, *42*(5), 776-782.

Requejo, A. M., Ortega, R. M., Robles, F., Navia, B., Faci, M., & Aparicio, A. (2003). Influence of nutrition on cognitive function in a group of elderly, independently living people. *European Journal of Clinical Nutrition*, *57*, S54-S57.

Morris, M. C., Evans, D. A., Tangney, C. C., Bienias, J. L., Schneider, J. A., Wilson, R. S., & Scherr, P. A. (2006). Dietary copper and high saturated and trans fat intakes associated with cognitive decline. *Archives of neurology*, *63*(8), 1085-1088.

Lee, Y., Back, J. H., Kim, J., Kim, S. H., Na, D. L., Cheong, H. K., ... & Kim, Y. G. (2010). Systematic review of health behavioral risks and cognitive health in older adults. *International psychogeriatrics*, *22*(2), 174-187.

Ye, X., Gao, X., Scott, T., & Tucker, K. L. (2011). Habitual sugar intake and cognitive function among middle-aged and older Puerto Ricans without diabetes. *British journal of nutrition*, *106*(9), 1423-1432.

Alosco, M. L., Spitznagel, M. B., Raz, N., Cohen, R., Sweet, L. H., Colbert, L. H., ... & Gunstad, J. (2013). Dietary habits moderate the association between heart failure and cognitive impairment. *Journal of nutrition in gerontology and geriatrics*, *32*(2), 106-121.

Okereke, O. I., Rosner, B. A., Kim, D. H., Kang, J. H., Cook, N. R., Manson, J. E., ... & Grodstein, F. (2012). Dietary fat types and 4-year cognitive change in community-dwelling older women. *Annals of neurology*, *72*(1), 124-134.

Wu, A., Ying, Z., & Gomez-Pinilla, F. (2004). The interplay between oxidative stress and brain-derived neurotrophic factor modulates the outcome of a saturated fat diet on synaptic plasticity and cognition. *European Journal of Neuroscience*, *19*(7), 1699-1707.

Bayer-Carter, J. L., Green, P. S., Montine, T. J., VanFossen, B., Baker, L. D., Watson, G. S., ... & Tsai, E. (2011). Diet intervention and cerebrospinal fluid biomarkers in amnestic mild cognitive impairment. *Archives of neurology*, *68*(6), 743-752.

Hao, S., Dey, A., Yu, X., & Stranahan, A. M. (2016). Dietary obesity reversibly induces synaptic stripping by microglia and impairs hippocampal plasticity. *Brain, behavior, and immunity*, *51*, 230-239.

Boitard, C., Cavaroc, A., Sauvant, J., Aubert, A., Castanon, N., Layé, S., & Ferreira, G. (2014). Impairment of hippocampal-dependent memory induced by juvenile high-fat diet intake is associated with enhanced hippocampal inflammation in rats. *Brain, behavior, and immunity*, *40*, 9-17.

Molteni, R., Barnard, R. J., Ying, Z., Roberts, C. K., & Gomez-Pinilla, F. (2002). A high-fat, refined sugar diet reduces hippocampal brain-derived neurotrophic factor, neuronal plasticity, and learning. *Neuroscience*, 112(4), 803-814.

Driving force No.2: trans fat

Hu, F. B., & Willett, W. C. (2002). Optimal diets for prevention of coronary heart disease. *Jama*, *288*(20), 2569-2578.

Mozaffarian, D., Aro, A., & Willett, W. C. (2009). Health effects of trans-fatty acids: experimental and observational evidence. *European journal of clinical nutrition*, *63*, S5-S21.

Dhibi, M., Brahmi, F., Mnari, A., Houas, Z., Chargui, I., Bchir, L., ... & Hammami, M. (2011). The intake of high fat diet with different trans fatty acid levels differentially induces oxidative stress and non alcoholic fatty liver disease (NAFLD) in rats. *Nutrition & metabolism*, *8*(1), 65.

Devore, E. E., Stampfer, M. J., Breteler, M. M., Rosner, B., Kang, J. H., Okereke, O., ... & Grodstein, F. (2009). Dietary fat intake and cognitive decline in women with type 2 diabetes. *Diabetes care*, *32*(4), 635-640.

Driving force No.3: refined sugars

Lowette, K., Roosen, L., Tack, J., & Berghe, P. V. (2015). Effects of high-fructose diets on central appetite signaling and cognitive function. *Frontiers in nutrition*, *2*.

Ludwig, D. S. (2007). Clinical update: the low-glycaemic-index diet. *The Lancet*, *369*(9565), 890-892.

Schwartz, D. L., Gilstad-Hayden, K., Carroll-Scott, A., Grilo, S. A., McCaslin, C., Schwartz, M., & Ickovics, J. R. (2015). Energy drinks and youth self-reported hyperactivity/inattention symptoms. *Academic pediatrics*, *15*(3), 297-304.

Scharf, R. J., & DeBoer, M. D. (2016). Sugar-sweetened beverages and children's health. *Annual review of public health*, 37, 273-293.

American Diabetes Association. *Glycemic Index and Diabetes*. Available at http://www.diabetes.org/food-and-fitness/ food/what-can-i-eat/understanding-carbohydrates/glycemic- index-and-diabetes.html?referrer=https://www.google.co.jp/ (last accessed 2017-12-16)

Sünram-Lea, S. I., & Owen, L. (2017). The impact of diet-based glycaemic response and glucose regulation on cognition: evidence across the lifespan. *Proceedings of the Nutrition Society*, *76*(4), 466-477.

For overweight and obesity, see Chapter 12 of Chen, C. (2017). *Plato's Insight: How Physical Exercise Boosts Mental Excellence*. London: Brain & Life Publishing

Driving force No.4: salt

Susic, D., & Frohlich, E. D. (2012). Salt consumption and cardiovascular, renal, and hypertensive diseases: clinical and mechanistic aspects. *Current opinion in lipidology*, *23*(1), 11-16.

Liu, Y. Z., Chen, J. K., Li, Z. P., Zhao, T., Ni, M., Li, D. J., ... & Shen, F. M. (2014). High-salt diet enhances hippocampal oxidative stress and cognitive impairment in mice. *Neurobiology of learning and memory*, 114, 10-15.

Afsar, B. (2013). The relationship between cognitive function, depressive behaviour and sleep quality with 24-h urinary sodium excretion in patients with essential hypertension. *High Blood Pressure & Cardiovascular Prevention*, *20*(1), 19-24.

Fiocco, A. J., Shatenstein, B., Ferland, G., Payette, H., Belleville, S., Kergoat, M. J., ... & Greenwood, C. E. (2012). Sodium intake and physical activity impact cognitive maintenance in older adults: the NuAge Study. *Neurobiology of aging*, *33*(4), 829-e21.

Stewart, M. W., Traylor, A. C., & Bratzke, L. C. (2015). Nutrition and cognition in older adults with heart failure: a systematic review. *Journal of gerontological nursing*, *41*(11), 50-59.

Gorelick, P. B., Scuteri, A., Black, S. E., DeCarli, C., Greenberg, S. M., Iadecola, C., ... & Petersen, R. C. (2011). Vascular contributions to cognitive impairment and dementia. *Stroke*, *42*(9), 2672-2713.

Chapter 12. The Case for Dairy

Hess, J. M., Jonnalagadda, S. S., & Slavin, J. L. (2016). Dairy foods: current evidence of their effects on bone, cardiometabolic, cognitive, and digestive health. *Comprehensive Reviews in Food Science and Food Safety*, *15*(2), 251-268.

Fat-free or low-fat dairy reliably enhances cognitive functions

Kim, S. H., Kim, W. K., & Kang, M. H. (2016). Relationships between milk consumption and academic performance, learning motivation and strategy, and personality in Korean adolescents. *Nutrition research and practice*, *10*(2), 198-205.

Wu, L., & Sun, D. (2016). Meta-Analysis of Milk Consumption and the Risk of Cognitive Disorders. *Nutrients*, 8(12), 824.

Crichton, G. E., Bryan, J., Murphy, K. J., & Buckley, J. (2010). Review of dairy consumption and cognitive performance in adults: findings and methodological issues. *Dementia and geriatric cognitive disorders*, *30*(4), 352-361.

Research with insignificant or negative findings

Kesse-Guyot, E., Assmann, K. E., Andreeva, V. A., Ferry, M., Hercberg, S., Galan, P., & SU. VI. MAX 2 Research Group. (2016). Consumption of dairy products and cognitive functioning: Findings from the SU. VI. MAX 2 study. *The journal of nutrition, health & aging*, *20*(2), 128-137.

Petruski-Ivleva, N. (2017). *The Association of Habitual Milk Intake with the Rate of Cognitive Decline, and Risk of Mild Cognitive Impairment and Dementia* (Doctoral dissertation, The University of North Carolina at Chapel Hill).

Crichton, G. E., Murphy, K. J., & Bryan, J. (2010). Dairy intake and cognitive health in middle-aged South Australians. *Asia Pacific journal of clinical nutrition, 19*(2), 161-171.

Crichton, G. E., Murphy, K. J., Howe, P. R., Buckley, J. D., & Bryan, J. (2012). Dairy consumption and working memory performance in overweight and obese adults. *Appetite, 59*(1), 34-40.

Chronic disease

Pei, R., Martin, D. A., DiMarco, D. M., & Bolling, B. W. (2017). Evidence for the effects of yogurt on gut health and obesity. *Critical reviews in food science and nutrition, 57*(8), 1569-1583.

Drouin-Chartier, J. P., Brassard, D., Tessier-Grenier, M., Côté, J. A., Labonté, M. È., Desroches, S., ... & Lamarche, B. (2016). Systematic review of the association between dairy product consumption and risk of cardiovascular-related clinical outcomes. *Advances in Nutrition: An International Review Journal, 7*(6), 1026-1040.

Pasin, G., & Comerford, K. B. (2015). Dairy foods and dairy proteins in the management of type 2 diabetes: A systematic review of the clinical evidence. *Advances in Nutrition: An International Review Journal, 6*(3), 245-259.

Three cups of fat-free or low-fat dairy per day

US Department of Health and Human Services. (2015). 2015–2020 dietary guidelines for Americans. *Washington (DC): USDA.*

Yogurt and gut microbiota

Fisberg, M., & Machado, R. (2015). History of yogurt and current patterns of consumption. *Nutrition reviews, 73*(suppl_1), 4-7.

Niv, M., Levy, W., & Greenstein, N. M. (1963). Yogurt in the treatment of infantile diarrhea. *Clinical Pediatrics, 2*(7), 407-411.

Pashapour, N., & Iou, S. G. (2006). Evaluation of yogurt effect on acute diarrhea in 6-24-month-old hospitalized infants. *The Turkish journal of pediatrics, 48*(2), 115.

Stecher, B., & Hardt, W. D. (2011). Mechanisms controlling pathogen colonization of the gut. *Current opinion in microbiology, 14*(1), 82-91.

Brown, K., DeCoffe, D., Molcan, E., & Gibson, D. L. (2012). Diet-induced dysbiosis of the intestinal microbiota and the effects on immunity and disease. *Nutrients, 4*(8), 1095-1119.

Mckinley, M. C. (2005). The nutrition and health benefits of yoghurt. *International journal of dairy technology, 58*(1), 1-12.

Cryan, J. F., & Dinan, T. G. (2012). Mind-altering microorganisms: the impact of the gut microbiota on brain and behaviour. *Nature reviews neuroscience*, *13*(10), 701-712.

Collins, S. M., Surette, M., & Bercik, P. (2012). The interplay between the intestinal microbiota and the brain. *Nature Reviews Microbiology*, *10*(11), 735-742.

De Vadder, F., Kovatcheva-Datchary, P., Goncalves, D., Vinera, J., Zitoun, C., Duchampt, A., ... & Mithieux, G. (2014). Microbiota-generated metabolites promote metabolic benefits via gut-brain neural circuits. *Cell*, *156*(1), 84-96.

Dinan, T. G., Stilling, R. M., Stanton, C., & Cryan, J. F. (2015). Collective unconscious: how gut microbes shape human behavior. *Journal of psychiatric research*, *63*, 1-9.

Forsyth, C. B., Farhadi, A., Jakate, S. M., Tang, Y., Shaikh, M., & Keshavarzian, A. (2009). Lactobacillus GG treatment ameliorates alcohol-induced intestinal oxidative stress, gut leakiness, and liver injury in a rat model of alcoholic steatohepatitis. *Alcohol*, *43*(2), 163-172.

Davari, S., Talaei, S. A., & Alaei, H. (2013). Probiotics treatment improves diabetes-induced impairment of synaptic activity and cognitive function: behavioral and electrophysiological proofs for microbiome–gut–brain axis. *Neuroscience*, *240*, 287-296.

Kim, B., Hong, V. M., Yang, J., Hyun, H., Im, J. J., Hwang, J., ... & Kim, J. E. (2016). A review of fermented foods with beneficial effects on brain and cognitive function. *Preventive nutrition and food science*, *21*(4), 297.

Brown, A. C., & Valiere, A. (2004). Probiotics and medical nutrition therapy. *Nutrition in clinical care: an official publication of Tufts University*, *7*(2), 56.

Chapter 13. Spices, as Precious as Gold

Quote Columbus available at https://history.hanover.edu/ courses/excerpts/111columbus.html (last accessed 2017-12-19)

Spices are powerful antioxidants

Kochhar, K. P. (2008). Dietary spices in health and diseases: I. *Indian J Physiol Pharmacol*, 52(2), 106-122.

Paur, I., Carlsen, M. H., Halvorsen, B. L., & Blomhoff, R. (2011). Antioxidants in Herbs and Spices: Roles in Oxidative Stress and Redox Signaling. In: Benzie IFF, Wachtel-Galor S, editors. *Herbal Medicine: Biomolecular and Clinical Aspects*. 2nd edition. Boca Raton (FL): CRC Press/Taylor & Francis; 2011. Chapter 2.

Kris-Etherton, P. M., Hecker, K. D., Bonanome, A., Coval, S. M., Binkoski, A. E., Hilpert, K. F., ... & Etherton, T. D. (2002). Bioactive compounds in foods: their role in the prevention of cardiovascular disease and cancer. *The American journal of medicine*, *113*(9), 71-88.

Warshafsky, S., Kamer, R. S., & Sivak, S. L. (1993). Effect of Garlic on Total Serum CholesterolA Meta-Analysis. *Annals of internal medicine*, *119*(7_Part_1), 599-605.

Stevinson, C., Pittler, M. H., & Ernst, E. (2000). Garlic for Treating HypercholesterolemiaA Meta-Analysis of Randomized Clinical Trials. *Annals of internal medicine*, *133*(6), 420-429.

Rahman, K. (2003). Garlic and aging: new insights into an old remedy. *Ageing research reviews*, 2(1), 39-56.

Howes, M. J. R., & Houghton, P. J. (2003). Plants used in Chinese and Indian traditional medicine for improvement of memory and cognitive function. *Pharmacology Biochemistry and Behavior*, 75(3), 513-527.

Islam, A., Saif Khandker, S., Alam, F., Ibrahim Khalil, M., Amjad Kamal, M., & Hua Gan, S. (2017). Alzheimer's Disease and Natural Products: Future Regimens Emerging from Nature. *Current topics in medicinal chemistry*, *17*(12), 1408-1428.

Carlsen, M. H., Halvorsen, B. L., Holte, K., Bøhn, S. K., Dragland, S., Sampson, L., ... & Barikmo, I. (2010). The total antioxidant content of more than 3100 foods, beverages, spices, herbs and supplements used worldwide. *Nutrition journal*, *9*(1), 3.

Pellegrini, N., Serafini, M., Salvatore, S., Del Rio, D., Bianchi, M., & Brighenti, F. (2006). Total antioxidant capacity of spices, dried fruits, nuts, pulses, cereals and sweets consumed in Italy assessed by three different in vitro assays. *Molecular nutrition & food research*, *50*(11), 1030-1038.

Lu, M., Yuan, B., Zeng, M., & Chen, J. (2011). Antioxidant capacity and major phenolic compounds of spices commonly consumed in China. *Food Research International*, *44*(2), 530-536.

Garlic, ginger, and cognitive functions in animal research

Modi, K. K., Roy, A., Brahmachari, S., Rangasamy, S. B., & Pahan, K. (2015). Cinnamon and its metabolite sodium benzoate attenuate the activation of p21rac and protect memory and learning in an animal model of Alzheimer's disease. *PloS one*, *10*(6), e0130398.

Subedee, L., Suresh, R. N., Jayanthi, M. K., Kalabharathi, H. L., Satish, A. M., & Pushpa, V. H. (2015). Preventive role of Indian black pepper in animal models of Alzheimer's disease. *Journal of clinical and diagnostic research: JCDR*, *9*(4), FF01.

Borek, C. (2006). Garlic reduces dementia and heart-disease risk. *The Journal of nutrition*, *136*(3), 810S-812S.

Nishiyama, N., Moriguchi, T., & Saito, H. (1997). Beneficial effects of aged garlic extract on learning and memory impairment in the senescence-accelerated mouse. *Experimental gerontology*, *32*(1), 149-160.

Moriguchi, T., Saito, H., & Nishiyama, N. (1997). Anti-ageing effect of aged garlic extract in the inbred brain atrophy mouse model. *Clinical and experimental pharmacology and physiology, 24*(3-4), 235-242.

Chauhan, N. B., & Sandoval, J. (2007). Amelioration of early cognitive deficits by aged garlic extract in Alzheimer's transgenic mice. *Phytotherapy Research, 21*(7), 629-640.

Nillert, N., Pannangrong, W., Welbat, J. U., Chaijaroonkhanarak, W., Sripanidkulchai, K., & Sripanidkulchai, B. (2017). Neuroprotective Effects of Aged Garlic Extract on Cognitive Dysfunction and Neuroinflammation Induced by β-Amyloid in Rats. *Nutrients, 9*(1), 24.

Ali, B. H., Blunden, G., Tanira, M. O., & Nemmar, A. (2008). Some phytochemical, pharmacological and toxicological properties of ginger (Zingiber officinale Roscoe): a review of recent research. *Food and chemical Toxicology, 46*(2), 409-420.

Oboh, G., Ademiluyi, A. O., & Akinyemi, A. J. (2012). Inhibition of acetylcholinesterase activities and some pro-oxidant induced lipid peroxidation in rat brain by two varieties of ginger (Zingiber officinale). *Experimental and toxicologic pathology, 64*(4), 315-319.

Adolphus, K., Lawton, C. L., Champ, C. L., & Dye, L. (2016). The effects of breakfast and breakfast composition on cognition in children and adolescents: a systematic review. *Advances in Nutrition: An International Review Journal, 7*(3), 590S-612S.

Blake, D. T., Terry, A. V., Plagenhoef, M., Constantinidis, C., & Liu, R. (2017). Potential for intermittent stimulation of nucleus basalis of meynert to impact treatment of alzheimer's disease. *Communicative & Integrative Biology*, *27*(just-accepted), 00-00.

Francis, P.T. (2005). The interplay of neurotransmitters in Alzheimer's disease. *CNS Spectr*. 10(11 Suppl 18):6-9.

Korni, F. M. M., & Khalil, F. (2017). Effect of ginger and its nanoparticles on growth performance, cognition capability, immunity and prevention of motile Aeromonas septicaemia in Cyprinus carpio fingerlings. *Aquaculture Nutrition*.

Karam, A., Nadia, A., Abd, E. F., Nemat, A., & Siham, M. A. E. S. (2014). Protective effect of ginger (Zingiber officinale) on Alzheimer's disease induced in rats. *J Neuroinfect Dis*, *5*(159), 2.

Lim, S., Moon, M., Oh, H., Kim, H. G., Kim, S. Y., & Oh, M. S. (2014). Ginger improves cognitive function via NGF-induced ERK/CREB activation in the hippocampus of the mouse. *The Journal of nutritional biochemistry*, *25*(10), 1058-1065.

Turmeric and curry

Prasad, S., & Aggarwal, B. B. (2011). Turmeric, the golden spice: From Traditional Medicine to Modern Medicine. In: Benzie IFF, Wachtel-Galor S, editors. *Herbal Medicine: Biomolecular and Clinical Aspects*. 2nd edition. Boca Raton (FL): CRC Press/Taylor & Francis; 2011. Chapter 13.

Xu, Y., Ku, B., Tie, L., Yao, H., Jiang, W., Ma, X., & Li, X. (2006). Curcumin reverses the effects of chronic stress on behavior, the HPA axis, BDNF expression and phosphorylation of CREB. *Brain research, 1122*(1), 56-64.

Zhang, Y., Han, M., Liu, Z., Wang, J., He, Q., & Liu, J. (2012). Chinese herbal formula xiao yao san for treatment of depression: a systematic review of randomized controlled trials. *Evidence-Based Complementary and Alternative Medicine, 2012*.

Ng, T. P., Chiam, P. C., Lee, T., Chua, H. C., Lim, L., & Kua, E. H. (2006). Curry consumption and cognitive function in the elderly. *American journal of epidemiology, 164*(9), 898-906.

Potter, P. E. (2013). Curcumin: a natural substance with potential efficacy in Alzheimer's disease. *Journal of experimental Pharmacology, 5*, 23.

Mishra, S., & Palanivelu, K. (2008). The effect of curcumin (turmeric) on Alzheimer's disease: An overview. *Annals of Indian Academy of Neurology, 11*(1), 13.

Ganguli, M., Chandra, V., Kamboh, M. I., Johnston, J. M., Dodge, H. H., Thelma, B. K., ... & DeKosky, S. T. (2000). Apolipoprotein E polymorphism and Alzheimer disease: the Indo-US cross-national dementia study. *Archives of Neurology, 57*(6), 824-830.

Chapter 14. Mood-boosting Foods

Feelings, or moods, are the output of the brain

Hodes, G. E., Kana, V., Menard, C., Merad, M., & Russo, S. J. (2015). Neuroimmune mechanisms of depression. *Nature neuroscience*, *18*(10), 1386-1393.

Fenton, W. S., & Stover, E. S. (2006). Mood disorders: cardiovascular and diabetes comorbidity. *Current Opinion in Psychiatry*, *19*(4), 421-427.

Maes, M., Kubera, M., Obuchowiczwa, E., Goehler, L., & Brzeszcz, J. (2011). Depression's multiple comorbidities explained by (neuro) inflammatory and oxidative & nitrosative stress pathways. *Neuroendocrinol Lett*, *32*(1), 7-24.

The healthy food patterns for feelings

Molendijk, M., Molero, P., Sánchez-Pedreño, F. O., Van der Does, W., & Martínez-González, M. A. (2017). Diet quality and depression risk: a systematic review and dose-response meta-analysis of prospective studies. *Journal of affective disorders*.

Marx W, Moseley G, Berk M, Jacka F. (2017) Nutritional psychiatry: the present state of the evidence. *Proc Nutr Soc*. 2017 Sep 25:1-10. doi: 10.1017/S0029665117002026.

Li, Y., Lv, M. R., Wei, Y. J., Sun, L., Zhang, J. X., Zhang, H. G., & Li, B. (2017). Dietary patterns and depression risk: A meta-analysis. *Psychiatry Research*.

O'Neil, A., Quirk, S. E., Housden, S., Brennan, S. L., Williams, L. J., Pasco, J. A., ... & Jacka, F. N. (2014). Relationship between diet and mental health in children and adolescents: a systematic review. *American journal of public health*, *104*(10), e31-e42.

Lang, U. E., Beglinger, C., Schweinfurth, N., Walter, M., & Borgwardt, S. (2015). Nutritional aspects of depression. *Cellular Physiology and Biochemistry*, *37*(3), 1029-1043.

Experiments

McMillan, L., Owen, L., Kras, M., & Scholey, A. (2011). Behavioural effects of a 10-day Mediterranean diet. Results from a pilot study evaluating mood and cognitive performance. *Appetite*, *56*(1), 143-147.

Lee, J., Pase, M., Pipingas, A., Raubenheimer, J., Thurgood, M., Villalon, L., ... & Scholey, A. (2015). Switching to a 10-day Mediterranean-style diet improves mood and cardiovascular function in a controlled crossover study. *Nutrition*, *31*(5), 647-652.

Jacka, F. N., O'Neil, A., Opie, R., Itsiopoulos, C., Cotton, S., Mohebbi, M., ... & Brazionis, L. (2017). A randomised controlled trial of dietary improvement for adults with major depression (the 'SMILES'trial). *BMC medicine*, *15*(1), 23.

Sánchez-Villegas, A., Martínez-González, M. A., Estruch, R., Salas-Salvadó, J., Corella, D., Covas, M. I., ... & Pintó, X.

(2013). Mediterranean dietary pattern and depression: the PREDIMED randomized trial. *BMC medicine*, *11*(1), 208.

Surveys

Ford, P. A., Jaceldo-Siegl, K., Lee, J. W., Youngberg, W., & Tonstad, S. (2013). Intake of Mediterranean foods associated with positive affect and low negative affect. *Journal of psychosomatic research*, *74*(2), 142-148.

Costarelli, V., Koretsi, E., & Georgitsogianni, E. (2013). Health-related quality of life of Greek adolescents: the role of the Mediterranean diet. *Quality of life research*, *22*(5), 951-956.

Landaeta-Díaz, L., Fernández, J. M., Silva-Grigoletto, M. D., Rosado-Alvarez, D., Gómez-Garduño, A., Gómez-Delgado, F., ... & Fuentes-Jiménez, F. (2013). Mediterranean diet, moderate-to-high intensity training, and health-related quality of life in adults with metabolic syndrome. *European journal of preventive cardiology*, *20*(4), 555-564.

Munoz, M. A., Fíto, M., Marrugat, J., Covas, M. I., & Schröder, H. (2008). Adherence to the Mediterranean diet is associated with better mental and physical health. *British Journal of Nutrition*, *101*(12), 1821-1827.

Psaltopoulou, T., Sergentanis, T. N., Panagiotakos, D. B., Sergentanis, I. N., Kosti, R., & Scarmeas, N. (2013). Mediterranean diet, stroke, cognitive impairment, and depression: a meta-analysis. *Annals of neurology*, *74*(4), 580-591.

The unhealthy food pattern for feelings

Lang, U. E., Beglinger, C., Schweinfurth, N., Walter, M., & Borgwardt, S. (2015). Nutritional aspects of depression. *Cellular Physiology and Biochemistry, 37*(3), 1029-1043.

Sánchez-Villegas, A., Verberne, L., De Irala, J., Ruíz-Canela, M., Toledo, E., Serra-Majem, L., & Martínez-González, M. A. (2011). Dietary fat intake and the risk of depression: the SUN Project. *PloS one, 6*(1), e16268.

Sánchez-Villegas, A., Toledo, E., de Irala, J., Ruiz-Canela, M., Pla-Vidal, J., & Martínez-González, M. A. (2012). Fast-food and commercial baked goods consumption and the risk of depression. *Public health nutrition, 15*(3), 424-432.

Saunders, P. A., Copeland, J. R., Dewey, M. E., Davidson, I. A., McWilliam, C., Sharma, V., & Sullivan, C. (1991). Heavy drinking as a risk factor for depression and dementia in elderly men. Findings from the Liverpool longitudinal community study. *The British Journal of Psychiatry, 159*(2), 213-216.

House, J., DeVoe, S. E., & Zhong, C. B. (2014). Too impatient to smell the roses: exposure to fast food impedes happiness. *Social Psychological and Personality Science, 5*(5), 534-541.

Davis, J. F., Tracy, A. L., Schurdak, J. D., Tschöp, M. H., Lipton, J. W., Clegg, D. J., & Benoit, S. C. (2008). Exposure to elevated levels of dietary fat attenuates psychostimulant reward and mesolimbic dopamine turnover in the rat. *Behavioral neuroscience, 122*(6), 1257.

Knutson, B., Adams, C. M., Fong, G. W., & Hommer, D. (2001). Anticipation of increasing monetary reward selectively recruits nucleus accumbens. *Journal of Neuroscience*, *21*(16), RC159-RC159.

The case against comfort food

Park, C. (2004). Efficient or enjoyable? Consumer values of eating-out and fast food restaurant consumption in Korea. *International Journal of Hospitality Management*, *23*(1), 87-94.

Dallman, M. F., Pecoraro, N. C., & la Fleur, S. E. (2005). Chronic stress and comfort foods: self-medication and abdominal obesity. *Brain, behavior, and immunity*, *19*(4), 275-280.

Macht, M., & Mueller, J. (2007). Interactive effects of emotional and restrained eating on responses to chocolate and affect. *The Journal of nervous and mental disease*, *195*(12), 1024-1026.

Kandiah, J., Yake, M., Jones, J., & Meyer, M. (2006). Stress influences appetite and comfort food preferences in college women. *Nutrition Research*, *26*(3), 118-123.

Ortolani, D., Oyama, L. M., Ferrari, E. M., Melo, L. L., & Spadari-Bratfisch, R. C. (2011). Effects of comfort food on food intake, anxiety-like behavior and the stress response in rats. *Physiology & behavior*, *103*(5), 487-492.

Wansink, B., Cheney, M. M., & Chan, N. (2003). Exploring comfort food preferences across age and gender. *Physiology & behavior*, *79*(4), 739-747.

Dubé, L., LeBel, J. L., & Lu, J. (2005). Affect asymmetry and comfort food consumption. *Physiology & Behavior*, *86*(4), 559-567.

Epel, E., Jimenez, S., Brownell, K., Stroud, L., Stoney, C., & Niaura, R. A. Y. (2004). Are stress eaters at risk for the metabolic syndrome?. *Annals of the New York Academy of Sciences*, *1032*(1), 208-210.

Macht, M., & Dettmer, D. (2006). Everyday mood and emotions after eating a chocolate bar or an apple. *Appetite*, 46, 332e336.

Parker, G., Parker, I., & Brotchie, H. (2006). Mood state effects of chocolate. *Journal of affective disorders*, *92*(2), 149-159.

Tan, C. C., & Holub, S. C. (2018). The effects of happiness and sadness on Children's snack consumption. *Appetite*.

Yeomans, M. R. (2017). Adverse effects of consuming high fat–sugar diets on cognition: implications for understanding obesity. *Proceedings of the Nutrition Society*, 1-11.

Chapter 15. Foods That Help You Sleep

The function of sleep in a healthy brain

Rasch, B., & Born, J. (2013). About sleep's role in memory. *Physiological reviews*, *93*(2), 681-766.

Xie, L., Kang, H., Xu, Q., Chen, M. J., Liao, Y., Thiyagarajan, M., ... & Takano, T. (2013). Sleep drives metabolite clearance from the adult brain. *Science*, *342*(6156), 373-377.

Mawuenyega, K. G., Sigurdson, W., Ovod, V., Munsell, L., Kasten, T., Morris, J. C., ... & Bateman, R. J. (2010). Decreased clearance of CNS β-amyloid in Alzheimer's disease. *Science*, *330*(6012), 1774-1774.

The neurobiology of sleep

Claustrat, B., Brun, J., & Chazot, G. (2005). The basic physiology and pathophysiology of melatonin. *Sleep medicine reviews*, *9*(1), 11-24.

Ferracioli-Oda, E., Qawasmi, A., & Bloch, M. H. (2013). Meta-analysis: melatonin for the treatment of primary sleep disorders. *PloS one*, *8*(5), e63773.

Peuhkuri, K., Sihvola, N., & Korpela, R. (2012). Diet promotes sleep duration and quality. *Nutrition research*, *32*(5), 309-319.

Beydoun, M. A., Gamaldo, A. A., Canas, J. A., Beydoun, H. A., Shah, M. T., McNeely, J. M., & Zonderman, A. B. (2014). Serum nutritional biomarkers and their associations with sleep among US adults in recent national surveys. *PloS one*, *9*(8), e103490.

A healthy diet for thought is also a sleep diet

St-Onge, M. P., Mikic, A., & Pietrolungo, C. E. (2016). Effects of diet on sleep quality. *Advances in Nutrition: An International Review Journal, 7*(5), 938-949.

Katagiri, R., Asakura, K., Kobayashi, S., Suga, H., & Sasaki, S. (2014). Low intake of vegetables, high intake of confectionary, and unhealthy eating habits are associated with poor sleep quality among middle-aged female Japanese workers. *Journal of occupational health, 56*(5), 359-368.

Tan, X., Alén, M., Cheng, S. M., Mikkola, T. M., Tenhunen, J., Lyytikäinen, A., ... & Partinen, M. (2015). Associations of disordered sleep with body fat distribution, physical activity and diet among overweight middle-aged men. *Journal of sleep research, 24*(4), 414-424.

Papandreou, C. (2013). Independent associations between fatty acids and sleep quality among obese patients with obstructive sleep apnoea syndrome. *Journal of sleep research, 22*(5), 569-572.

Del Brutto, O. H., Mera, R. M., Ha, J. E., Gillman, J., Zambrano, M., & Castillo, P. R. (2016). Dietary fish intake and sleep quality: a population-based study. *Sleep medicine, 17*, 126-128.

Hansen, A. L., Dahl, L., Olson, G., Thornton, D., Graff, I. E., Frøyland, L., ... & Pallesen, S. (2014). Fish consumption, sleep, daily functioning, and heart rate variability. *Journal of clinical sleep medicine: JCSM: official publication of the American Academy of Sleep Medicine, 10*(5), 567.

Jaussent, I., Dauvilliers, Y., Ancelin, M. L., Dartigues, J. F., Tavernier, B., Touchon, J., ... & Besset, A. (2011). Insomnia symptoms in older adults: associated factors and gender differences. *The American Journal of Geriatric Psychiatry, 19*(1), 88-97.

St-Onge, M. P., Roberts, A., Shechter, A., & Choudhury, A. R. (2016). Fiber and saturated fat are associated with sleep arousals and slow wave sleep. *Journal of clinical sleep medicine: JCSM: official publication of the American Academy of Sleep Medicine, 12*(1), 19.

Bad foods that prevent you from a good night of sleep

Roehrs, T., & Roth, T. (2008). Caffeine: sleep and daytime sleepiness. *Sleep medicine reviews, 12*(2), 153-162.

Clark, I., and Landolt, H. P. (2017). Coffee, caffeine, and sleep: A systematic review of epidemiological studies and randomized controlled trials. *Sleep Med. Rev.* 31, 70–78

Unno, K., Noda, S., Kawasaki, Y., Yamada, H., Morita, A., Iguchi, K., & Nakamura, Y. (2017). Reduced Stress and Improved Sleep Quality Caused by Green Tea Are Associated with a Reduced Caffeine Content. *Nutrients, 9*(7), 777.

Roundtree, R. (2012). Insomnia: The impact on health and interventions to improve sleep. *Alternative and Complementary Therapies*, 18, 116–121

Masters, P. A. (2014). In the clinic: Insomnia. *Annals of Internal Medicine*, 161, ITC1–ITC14

Haario, P., Rahkonen, O., Laaksonen, M., Lahelma, E., & Lallukka, T. (2013). Bidirectional associations between insomnia symptoms and unhealthy behaviours. *Journal of sleep research*, *22*(1), 89-95.

Ebrahim, I. O., Shapiro, C. M., Williams, A. J., and Fenwick, P. B. (2013). Alcohol and sleep I: effects on normal sleep. *Alcohol. Clin. Exp. Res.* 37, 539–549.

Sleep diets: foods that promote sleep

Meng, X., Li, Y., Li, S., Zhou, Y., Gan, R. Y., Xu, D. P., & Li, H. B. (2017). Dietary Sources and Bioactivities of Melatonin. *Nutrients*, *9*(4), 367.

Peuhkuri, K., Sihvola, N., & Korpela, R. (2012). Diet promotes sleep duration and quality. *Nutrition research*, *32*(5), 309-319.

Knowlden, A. P., Hackman, C. L., & Sharma, M. (2016). Systematic Review of Dietary Interventions Targeting Sleep Behavior. *The Journal of Alternative and Complementary Medicine*, *22*(5), 349-362.

Valtonen, M. A. I. J. A., Niskanen, L., Kangas, A. P., & Koskinen, T. E. U. V. O. (2005). Effect of melatonin-rich night-time milk on sleep and activity in elderly institutionalized subjects. *Nordic journal of psychiatry*, *59*(3), 217-221.

Chen, W. Y., Giobbie-Hurder, A., Gantman, K., Savoie, J., Scheib, R., Parker, L. M., & Schernhammer, E. S. (2014). A randomized, placebo-controlled trial of melatonin on breast cancer survivors: impact on sleep, mood, and hot flashes. *Breast cancer research and treatment*, *145*(2), 381-388.

Campbell, A.N. (2015). A randomized placebo controlled trial of melatonin enriched milk—can it improve symptoms of insomnia? *Sleep*. 38:A232.

Bae, S. M., Jeong, J., Jeon, H. J., Bang, Y. R., & Yoon, I. Y. (2016). Effects of Melatonin-Rich Milk on Mild Insomnia Symptoms. *Sleep Medicine Research*, *7*(2), 60-67.

Yamamura, S., Morishima, H., Kumano-Go, T., Suganuma, N., Matsumoto, H., Adachi, H., ... & Takano, T. (2009). The effect of Lactobacillus helveticus fermented milk on sleep and health perception in elderly subjects. *European journal of clinical nutrition*, *63*(1), 100-105.

Takada, M., Nishida, K., Gondo, Y., Kikuchi-Hayakawa, H., Ishikawa, H., Suda, K., ... & Rokutan, K. (2017). Beneficial effects of Lactobacillus casei strain Shirota on academic stress-induced sleep disturbance in healthy adults: a double-blind, randomised, placebo-controlled trial. *Beneficial Microbes*, *8*(2), 153-162.

Pigeon, W. R., Carr, M., Gorman, C., & Perlis, M. L. (2010). Effects of a tart cherry juice beverage on the sleep of older adults with insomnia: a pilot study. *Journal of medicinal food*, 13(3), 579-583.

Howatson, G., Bell, P. G., Tallent, J., Middleton, B., Mchugh, M. P., & Ellis, J. (2012). Effect of tart cherry juice (Prunus cerasus) on melatonin levels and enhanced sleep quality. *European journal of nutrition*, *51*(8), 909-916.

Garrido, M., Paredes, S. D., Cubero, J., Lozano, M., Toribio-Delgado, A. F., Muñoz, J. L., ... & Rodríguez, A. B. (2010). Jerte Valley cherry-enriched diets improve nocturnal rest and increase 6-sulfatoxymelatonin and total antioxidant capacity in the urine of middle-aged and elderly humans. *Journals of Gerontology Series A: Biomedical Sciences and Medical Sciences*, *65*(9), 909-914.

Lin, H. H., Tsai, P. S., Fang, S. C., & Liu, J. F. (2011). Effect of kiwifruit consumption on sleep quality in adults with sleep problems. *Asia Pacific journal of clinical nutrition*, *20*(2), 169-174.

Chapter 16. We Are What We Eat

Vertumnus. Available https://en.wikipedia.org/wiki/Giuseppe_ Arcimboldo#/media/File:Vertumnus_%C3%A5rstidernas_gud _m%C3%A5lad_av_Guiseppe_Arcimboldo_1591_- _Skoklosters_slott_-_91503.tif (last accessed 2018-01-04)

Serafini M, Del Rio D, Yao DN, et al. (2011). Health Benefits of Tea. In: Benzie IFF, Wachtel-Galor S, editors. *Herbal Medicine: Biomolecular and Clinical Aspects*. 2nd edition. Boca Raton (FL): CRC Press/Taylor & Francis; Chapter 12.

INDEX

acetylcholine, 57, 85, 102

added sugar, 18, 19, 87, 97

adrenaline, 42, 57

aging, 16, 25, 40, 47, 63, 82, 90, 102

alcohol, 22, 25, 26, 27, 28, 29, 30, 31, 79, 118

amyloid, 25, 103, 114

antioxidant, 27, 30, 33, 41, 43, 44, 47, 52, 101, 102

attention, 3, 42, 43, 47, 50, 78, 91, 101

bacteria, 54, 65, 66, 97, 98, 99

BDNF, 17, 28, 43, 54, 57, 90, 98, 103

beer, 26, 29

berries, 40, 41, 43, 44, 52, 74, 101

beverage, 2, 20, 25, 28, 37, 41, 43, 70, 79, 87, 88, 91, 94, 110, 117

blood pressure, 92

caffeine, 33, 35, 36, 37, 117

cancer, 5, 24, 32, 33, 44, 55, 72, 76, 101

cardiovascular disease, 5, 22, 23, 24, 44, 55, 72, 76, 91, 92, 96, 101, 107

catechin, 11, 34, 35, 52

CHD, 22, 23, 26, 78, → coronary heart disease

chocolate, 2, 3, 4, 5, 6, 7, 9, 10, 17, 18, 19, 30, 36, 38, 46, 87, 88, 112, 123, 124, 126

cholesterol, 22, 26, 30, 85, 88

chronic diseases, 5, 9, 10, 22, 37, 44, 54, 55, 72, 75, 89, 111

cocoa, 9, 17, 18, 19, 36, 38, 46, 92

coffee, 36, 37, 38, 87, 117

cognitive, 5, 7, 10, 14, 16, 17, 19, 24, 25, 27, 34, 35, 37, 39, 40, 42, 43, 44, 47, 49, 50, 51, 52, 54, 55, 56,

57, 58, 59, 62, 63, 64, 65,
71, 75, 79, 82, 83, 84, 85,
87, 89, 90, 91, 92, 95, 96,
98, 99, 101, 102, 103,
107, 111, 114

cognitive decline, 16, 25,
37, 40, 42, 47, 48, 58, 63,
71, 75, 83, 87, 89, 90, 92,
95, 98

comfort food, 19, 93, 112,
113

coronary heart disease, 10,
22

dairy, 18, 79, 84, 85, 94, 95,
96, 97

dementia, 25, 26, 27, 58, 71,
84, 89, 107

depression, 107, 110

DHA, 56, 59, 60, 61, 62, 79,
120

diabetes, 5, 10, 55, 72, 91,
96, 98, 107

dietary fibers, 54, 98

dopamine, 42, 57, 90, 111

eggs, 79, 85, 118, 123

environmental challenge,
11, 14, 15, 16, 42, 53, 57,
109

EPA, 56, 59, 60, 61, 62, 79

executive function, 14, 87,
89

exercise, 8, 25, 107, 113

fast food, 88, 111, 112

fatigue, 118

fish, 56, 60, 61, 62, 63, 64,
65, 66, 71, 92, 109, 117,
118, 120

flavanol, 5, 11, 17, 18, 19,
20

fruit, 8, 25, 43, 44, 54, 68,
70, 71, 72, 73, 74, 75, 76,
77, 79, 109, 117, 118,
120, 124

glucose, 41, 81, 91

grapes, 25, 30, 43, 74, 118

green tea, 33, 34, 35, 36, 38,
46, 117, 124

growth factor, 13, 15, 17,
18, 28, 43, 54, 57, 82, 90,
98, 103, 106, 107

heaving drinking, 27

heavy drinking, 28, 118

hippocampus, 16, 36, 84,
90, 92

infection, 15, 42, 54, 101

inflammation, 13, 14, 15, 16, 18, 27, 42, 47, 57, 82, 85, 89, 92, 98, 106, 107

insomnia, 115, 117, 118

juice, 29, 30, 40, 44, 75, 87, 120, 124

junk food, 12, 15, 86, 93, 111, 123, 125

kiwifruit, 43, 44, 118, 120

legume, 52, 54, 69, 72

linguistic, 87, 89

lipoprotein, 26, 47

math, 63, 71, 95

Mediterranean diet, 46, 49, 50, 71, 78, 81, 82, 83, 84, 109, 110, 117, 124

melatonin, 44, 115, 116, 118, 119, 120

memory, 12, 14, 16, 27, 40, 41, 42, 48, 50, 57, 69, 84, 87, 90, 92, 96, 98, 102, 109, 114, 124

mild cognitive impairment, 37, 40, 85

milk, 18, 19, 94, 95, 96, 97, 99, 112, 118, 119, 123, 124

mineral, 30, 52, 61, 71, 79, 81, 84, 85, 94, 116

mortality, 23, 24, 37, 75, 76, 78

MUFA, 46, 47, 52, 59, 80, 88

neurogenesis, 107

neuron, 13, 14, 15, 16, 17, 18, 26, 27, 36, 42, 47, 56, 57, 82, 89, 92, 103, 106, 107

neurotransmission, 42, 69, 90, 98, 102, 107

Nobel Prize, 3, 4, 5, 6, 7, 8, 97, 123

Nurses' Health Study, 52

nuts, 50, 51, 52, 53, 54, 55, 56, 58, 59, 79, 92, 101, 110, 118, 124

obesity, 18, 98, 111, 113

olive oil, 45, 46, 47, 48, 49, 50, 59, 79, 80, 123

omega-3, 56, 57, 58, 59, 61, 65, 66, 71, 79

omega-6, 56, 57, 58

oxidative stress, 13, 15, 16, 18, 27, 41, 42, 47, 57, 58,

82, 85, 89, 90, 91, 92, 98, 106, 107

Parkinson's disease, 34, 107

polyphenol, 5, 11, 16, 17, 25, 26, 29, 30, 33, 34, 35, 38, 42, 43, 44, 46, 47, 48, 52, 53, 59, 71, 79, 101, 117

potassium, 72, 81, 94, 97

poultry, 79, 84, 124

processed meat, 79, 84, 85, 88, 110, 117

pro-inflammatory cytokine, 14, 16, 27, 47, 57, 89, 91

protein, 14, 18, 25, 52, 61, 71, 79, 84, 85, 88, 94, 103

PUFA, 56, 57, 58, 59, 61, 65, 66, 71

red meat, 69, 79, 84, 85, 124

refined grains, 80, 81

reward, 90, 111

ROS, 14, 16, 27, 42, 57

salt, 56, 88, 89, 92

saturated fat, 18, 19, 23, 46, 52, 56, 85, 88, 89, 90, 92,

95, 97, 110, 111, 112, 113

sausage, 85, 87, 111, 124

SCFA, 54

seafood, 59, 61, 62, 64, 65, 66, 69, 79, 123, 124, → fish

selenium, 61, 81

serotonin, 90

SFA, 46, 47, → saturated fat

snack, 70, 77, 124

socioeconomic, 25, 70

SOWING, 11, 12, 14, 15, 16, 18, 25, 28, 34, 42, 46, 57, 68, 70, 82, 89, 90, 107, 108

spatial, 16, 55, 89, 92, 98

spice, 79, 100, 101, 102, 123

spirits, 26, 28, 124

stress hormone, 13, 14, 15, 16, 18, 27, 42, 57, 82, 89, 98, 103, 106, 107, 109, 112

stroke, 10, 24, 76, 107

supplement, 42, 49, 50, 57, 58, 69, 102, 125

sweets, 19, 85, 88, 110, 112, 117, 124

Three-City Study, 47, 82

tomato, 43, 72, 73

trans fat, 88, 89, 90, 110

vegetable, 25, 43, 44, 54, 68, 69, 71, 72, 73, 75, 76, 77, 79, 99, 109, 117, 123, 124

vitamin, 28, 30, 42, 43, 44, 52, 59, 61, 71, 72, 79, 84, 85, 94, 97, 98, 116, 120

weight gain, 18, 53, 54

whole grains, 54, 79, 80, 81

wine, 21, 22, 23, 24, 25, 26, 29, 30, 38, 46, 51, 79, 80, 124

work performance, 12, 14, 15, 16, 18, 27, 34, 42, 47, 54, 57, 82, 85, 89, 90, 91, 92, 98, 103, 107

working memory, 14, 41, 50

yogurt, 79, 84, 94, 96, 97, 98, 123

zinc, 61, 84, 85, 94, 116

ABOUT THE AUTHOR

Dr. Chong Chen is a neuroscientist and possesses a Ph.D. in Medicine. Chong has authored 10 books, including two series called **The Anchor of Our Purest Thoughts** and **Your Baby's Developing Brain**.

As far as the future goes, Chong hopes that he will be able to translate scientific findings into ways that will allow regular people to live better lives. And through his books, he hopes that he can reach a much wider audience.

You can contact Chong and follow what he is writing about at: https://brainandlife.net

www.ingramcontent.com/pod-product-compliance
Lightning Source LLC
Chambersburg PA
CBHW022106280326
41933CB00007B/272